Dementia Care Training Manual for Staff Working in Nursing and Residential Settings

of related interest

Enriched Care Planning for People with Dementia
A Good Practice Guide for Delivering Person-Centred Care
Hazel May and Paul Edwards
ISBN 978 1 84310 405 6

The Pool Activity Level (PAL) Instrument for Occupational Profiling
A Practical Resource for Carers of People with Cognitive Impairment
3rd edition
Jackie Pool
ISBN 978 1 84310 594 7

Decision-Making, Personhood and Dementia
Exploring the Interface
Edited by Deborah O'Connor and Barbara Purves
ISBN 978 1 84310 585 5

Early Psychosocial Interventions in Dementia
Evidence-Based Practice
Moniz-Cook
ISBN 978 1 84310 683 8

Primary Care and Dementia
Steve Iliffe and Vari Drennan
Foreword by Murna Downs
ISBN 978 1 85302 997 4

The Activity Year Book
A Week by Week Guide for Use in Elderly Day and Residential Care
Anni Bowden and Nancy Lewthwaite
ISBN 978 1 84310 963 1

The Carer's Cosmetic Handbook
Simple Health and Beauty Tips for Older Persons
Sharon Tay
ISBN 978 1 84310 973 0

The Importance of Food and Mealtimes in Dementia Care
The Table is Set
Grethe Berg
Foreword by Aase-Marit Nygård
ISBN 978 1 84310 435 3

Dementia Care Training Manual for Staff Working in Nursing and Residential Settings

Danny Walsh

Jessica Kingsley Publishers
London and Philadelphia

First published in 2006
by Jessica Kingsley Publishers
116 Pentonville Road
London N1 9JB, UK
and
400 Market Street, Suite 400
Philadelphia, PA 19106, USA

www.jkp.com

Library of Congress Cataloging in Publication Data

Walsh, Danny.
  Dementia care training manual for staff working in nursing and residential settings / Danny Walsh. -- 1st American pbk. ed.
      p. ; cm.
  Includes bibliographical references and index.
  ISBN-13: 978-1-84310-318-9 (pbk. : alk. paper)
  ISBN-10: 1-84310-318-4 (pbk. : alk. paper) 1. Dementia--Patients--Care--Handbooks, manuals, etc.. 2. Caregivers--Handbooks, manuals, etc. I. Title.
  [DNLM: 1. Alzheimer Disease--Handbooks. 2. Health Personnel--education--Handbooks. 3. Homes for the Aged--organization & administration--Handbooks. 4. Residential Facilities--organization & administration--Handbooks. WT 39 W224d 2006]
  RC521.W35 2006
  362.196'831--dc22

                    2006010569

British Library Cataloguing in Publication Data
A CIP catalogue record for this book is available from the British Library

ISBN 978 1 84310 318 9

Contents

Photocopiable exercises and resources

List of Figures

Introduction

Care assistants in hospitals, nursing homes and other institutional settings have traditionally had the greatest daily contact with clients compared with other workers and professionals involved. In doing so they are called upon to show a range of skills which is as yet still greatly undervalued by society generally. Improving the quality of life of those suffering from the effects of dementia remains one of the hardest challenges facing today's caring professions. Despite this fact, care workers are among the lowest paid in British society and this reflects both a degree of ageism within society and an undervaluing of care work generally. Besides providing essential practical and physical hands-on care, working with clients who have dementia requires the use of skilled psychological techniques and social interventions for which carers seldom get the recognition they deserve.

This book provides a foundation of theory alongside practical guidelines and aims to empower care workers with the knowledge to make a real difference to the lives of the people for whom they are caring. It asks practitioners to reflect upon their own care by undertaking various exercises and asking questions of their own care environment and practice.

How to use this book

This book can be used either as a training manual for group sessions, or by individual carers to act as a focus for their learning. It is perhaps best used in groups as this fosters the sharing of ideas and reflection which can be so valuable in improving practice within a residential or nursing setting. You can work through it from beginning to end or use it as a dip-in resource. Practical exercises can be found at the end of each chapter; any of the exercises can be read and considered by an individual, but if you are using the book on your own you will find it helpful if you have a couple of colleagues who are willing to discuss them with you. When there is a tick symbol in the corner of the page, you can photocopy that page, so that you can give out copies to the members of your class, colleagues or discussion group. At the end of some sections there is a page where you can record your ideas for future reference.

I have linked each section to the relevant Training Organisation for the Personal Social Services (TOPSS) National Occupational Standards for Health and Social Care and the Mental Health Standards as many care workers will be working towards NVQs (National Vocational Qualifications).

There are several reasons why good dementia care is important:

- First, the number of people suffering from dementia is very large and rising. The Alzheimer's Society estimate that currently there are roughly 750,000 people in the UK with dementia, affecting five per cent of the over-65s and 20 per cent of the over-80s. The number of people surviving into old age is also increasing, which means that these figures will increase over the coming years. There are also approximately 18,000 people under 65 with dementia.

- Second, the nature of dementia underlines the importance of good care. Dementia is a devastating illness, which can strip away all abilities and leave the sufferer in a frightening world where they need total care. The ability to understand, communicate, eat, dress and toilet can all be lost; indeed all aspects of daily living can be affected. If we let it, it can destroy a person's dignity and individuality.

- Third, since there is still no cure for dementia, it is only good care practice which can make a real difference to the lives of sufferers. Indeed, most progress in the field of dementia care derives directly from improvements in care practice and a change in attitude towards dementia, taking a more positive outlook and providing clients with a good quality of life despite the disease.

There can be no hard-and-fast rules in dementia care, but there are strong underlying principles of good practice. The practices of care, for example, should be focused on whatever leads to a happy outcome for the client: providing sensory stimulation and human contact where cognitive ability has eliminated the possibility of conversation, for example. It is care workers who are in the best position to make a real positive impact. There should be recognition of the client as an equal, a fellow human, who is capable of experiencing pain and pleasure, of forming relationships and of being happy. In one sense the mission for carers is to find a way to make people happy in their dementia, to give the client back a sense of being a real person rather than just a dementia sufferer.

National Occupational Standards for Health and Social Care, Care Homes for Older People: National Minimum Standards, National Service Framework for Older People, and the Mental Health Standards Framework

Many of the chapters in this book will have direct links to aspects of these four important benchmarks. The specific links with National Occupational Standards, the Mental Health Standards and Care Home Standards will be highlighted at the end of each relevant chapter.

The National Occupational Standards for Health and Social Care

These form the basis for many NVQs, nationally recognised qualifications that show you are able to work to those standards. These standards for health and social care are written by TOPSS and denote what is considered to be 'best practice'. The standards are broken down into units and NVQs are gained by achieving groups of these units. Certain units are mandatory as these are seen as essential foundation skills. They are work-based qualifications: you are assessed on the job by assessors who observe you and discuss your understanding of your many roles and tasks. NVQs move through five levels, from Level 1, where you work under close supervision, to Levels 4 and 5, which require you to undertake much more responsibility, autonomy, management and often supervision of others. You collect evidence as to your competence in each unit and when you have satisfied your assessor in all the units you are awarded your NVQ.

Care Homes for Older People: National Minimum Standards

This is a statement of the national minimum standards for care homes that provide health or personal care for older people. The standards cover choice of home, health and personal care, daily life and social activities, complaints and protection, environmental standards, staffing and management issues. Among these are such important areas as privacy and dignity, client involvement, medication, social contact, autonomy and choice. It is hoped that the standards will foster an individualised approach to care in care homes. Whilst the standards themselves are not enforceable they are taken into account by care home inspections against the Care Homes Regulations 2001. The standards are written as care outcomes for service users and prefaced by a statement of good practice. Taken as a whole they provide a good guide to best practice and a useful audit tool.

National Service Framework for Older People

This forms part of the Government's NHS Plan and Social Service Improvement Programme. National service frameworks set national standards with a view to improving the quality of care and reducing national variations. The standard relates to all older people, whether they live at home, are in care or are in hospital. The aim is to ensure high-quality treatment that is individualised, dignified and respectful. The National Service Framework for Older People (Department of Health 2001) is broken down into eight major standards:

1. *Rooting out discrimination* – Age should not be a barrier to receiving services.

2. *Person centred care* – Focuses upon the need for individuality and choice.

3. *Intermediate care* – A new range of services to prevent unnecessary admission to long-term care or hospital admission and foster early discharge.

4. *General hospital care* – Highlights the need for specialist services and staff.

5. *Strokes* – Stroke prevention measures and specialist stroke service.

6. *Falls* – Measures to prevent falls and provide specialist treatment.

7. *Mental health* – Measures to provide better integrated services in this area.

8. *Health promotion* – Promoting active healthy life in old age.

Mental Health Standards Framework

Under the auspices of the Department of Health the employer-led consortium 'Skills for Health' published its first Mental Health Standards in 2003. It outlines the required standards for competencies for all those working within mental health settings. Many of the competencies have relevance to those working in the community with younger people with acute mental health problems. However, a good proportion relate to those working with dementia in nursing and residential home settings.

Further reading and references

Department of Health (2001) *National Service Framework for Older People – Modern Standards and Service Models.* London: DOH.

Department of Health (2002) *Care Homes for Older People: National Minimum Standards.* London: The Stationery Office.

Journal of Dementia Care. London: Hawker Publications. Available at www.careinfo.org

This has excellent articles too numerous to mention covering every aspect of dementia care and innovations in practice.

Skills for Health (2003) *Mental Health National Occupational Standards.* Available at www.skillsforhealth.org.uk

TOPSS (Training Organisation for the Personal Social Services) (2005) *Health and Social Care: National Occupational Standards. Unit and Element Titles and Numbers of the Reviewed National Occupational Standards and Qualifications. TOPSS England Final Edition.* February. Leeds: TOPSS.

Chapter 1
What is Dementia?

Key message

We are all individuals and dementia will affect us all differently. So, while we can look at core symptoms and behaviours that might be common in dementia, each individual will be affected and react in different ways. Each sufferer will retain a large element of their individuality and it is this which we need to latch on to and focus on in our interactions. There has been much poor care, the practitioners of which have seen sufferers merely as people with dementia for whom little can be done. What we need to try and do is to look beyond the label 'dementia' and try to get a sense of the individual beneath.

'Dementia' is a term used to describe a group of brain disorders which have a profound effect upon people's lives and which share similar symptoms. There are different types, as outlined below, but whatever its form, dementia will usually impact upon memory and orientation to time, place and person. This is frightening enough, but the ability to think and communicate can be also severely eroded. Mood and behaviour can be affected alongside a decline in the skills and abilities of everyday life. The cognitive impairment is such that someone with dementia cannot learn new information. Dementia persists over time and is irreversible. Eventually the person affected may come to need full-time nursing care.

Alzheimer's disease

The commonest form of dementia is Alzheimer's disease, accounting for about 55 per cent of all dementia cases. The disease is progressive and irreversible; it causes shrinkage of brain tissue and the death of brain cells. We do not know what causes it but we do know that changes in brain structure are linked to abnormalities with chromosome 21. Typically, the onset of Alzheimer's occurs when the person is in the mid-50s; however, it is not usually diagnosed until later when the effects are more noticeable. In the early stages of dementia the sufferer is often aware of their declining memory and cognitive functioning, which must be very frightening. Typically this insight leads to the sufferer denying problems and confabulating (making up stories or excuses to cover up the memory loss and errors); in this way it can be hard even for close family to pick up on the early signs. Women are more prone to Alzheimer's disease simply because they tend to live longer.

Vascular dementia

Vascular dementia is the second commonest form, caused by strokes in the brain where small blood vessels burst or become blocked. This cuts off the blood supply and therefore oxygen, causing the death of brain cells. It accounts for roughly 15 to 20 per cent of all dementia cases. The aspect of functioning that is affected depends on where the damage is in the brain, so there can be some aspects of mental functioning which are not affected. Unlike Alzheimer's disease the onset is often sudden, and may be followed by further strokes and further deterioration. This is usually called 'multi-infarct dementia' and it has a step-like progression, a sudden decline being followed by a period of stability (see Figure 1.1). Usually with each further stroke there is further decline.

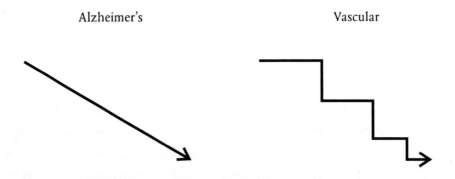

Alzheimer's   Vascular

Figure 1.1 Typical progression of Alzheimer's disease and vascular dementia

There may be several small unnoticed strokes which have the cumulative effect of damaging brain tissue sufficiently to cause dementia. Sufferers often have a high degree of insight in the early stages and this form of dementia is often accompanied by some physical loss of ability as a result of the stroke or strokes: typically, paralysis of limbs or loss of speech. Treatment is as for high blood pressure, which is factorial in causing strokes; thus, attention should be paid to diet and medication given to reduce blood pressure. Anti-coagulants can also be taken by sufferers to guard against the risk of a clot, and it is important that they stop smoking and reduce excessive alcohol intake, both of which are high risk factors for strokes.

Lewy body dementia

In Lewy body dementia small bodies grow in and destroy nerve cells in the brain; it accounts for around 15 to 20 per cent of all dementias. Typically, language, concentration and coordination are affected, with falls being a common occurrence. The loss of memory that is usually associated with a dementia is not so common among sufferers with Lewy body dementia and there is also some fluctuation between periods of lucidity and confusion. Auditory and visual hallucinations are common.

Creutzfeldt–Jakob disease

More commonly known as 'Mad cow disease', Creutzfeldt–Jakob disease, or CJD, has a rapid onset and causes rapid decline. It can occur at any age; it is especially tragic when it affects younger people. It is transmitted by eating beef infected with BSE. The symptoms occur some years after infection and the result is a full dementia. The epidemic of CJD which was at first expected failed to materialise and there are only some 200 cases worldwide; however, there may be more to come.

Pick's disease

Pick's disease is said to account for about five per cent of all dementias and women are twice as likely as men to suffer from it. It affects the frontal lobes of the brain and progresses slowly. It gives rise to profound personality changes which often manifest as disinhibited and inappropriate behaviour. This occurs alongside a deterioration in speech and eventual memory decline.

Depressive pseudo dementia

Often it can be very difficult to tell the early stages of dementia from depression, hence the name 'pseudo dementia'. Both dementia and depression are characterised by poor concentration, poor memory, withdrawal and low scores on cognitive tests. In cases of dementia, however, the symptoms persist over time and do not respond to anti-depressant medication; the sufferer will often have a go at an activity and be unaware that they are doing it wrong. Sufferers from depression, on the other hand, will often undertake the activity slowly and give up due to lack of motivation.

Rarer dementias

People in the later stages of suffering the AIDS virus can also succumb to a dementia, as can some people in the latter stages of Parkinson's disease. Sufferers of Down's Syndrome can also develop a progressive form of dementia similar to Alzheimer's in their middle age. Down's Syndrome is associated with an extra chromosome 21, so this is an important area for further research. Huntington's Chorea is a rare degenerative brain disorder which is inherited and affects half of all offspring. Tragically it is not usually noticed until the sufferer has reached their early 30s by which time most people have started a family. It is characterised by incapacitating jerking movements of the limbs and is usually accompanied by a form of dementia. Long-term misuse of alcohol can cause a dementia known as Korsakov's Syndrome which is typified by an extremely short memory span. It is caused by a deficiency of the B vitamin thiamine.

Acute confusional state and other causes

Chest and urine infections can cause confusional states which mimic dementia but are all treatable with antibiotics. Constipation is also one of the biggest causes of confusion in older people, but is often overlooked. Other common reasons for confusion are pain, the side effects of medication, poor fluid intake, alcohol, brain tumour, grief and depression. This list is not exhaustive and it demonstrates the need for a thorough initial screening and assessment process.

Reminder

Dementia is not a part of the normal ageing process. There is some cognitive and intellectual decline which can be put down to normal ageing, but dementia is a terminal illness that has a far greater impact upon the individual. Accurate estimates that one in five people over 80 will suffer dementia can make old age seem like a depressing scenario and if we work with older people with dementia we can get a jaundiced and negative view of the future. Thus we should recognise the fact that 80 per cent of the over 80s will *not* suffer dementia.

Further reading and references

Cheston, R. and Bender, M. (1999) *Understanding Dementia: The Man with the Worried Eyes*. London: Jessica Kingsley Publishers.

Chapter 2, 'The present formulation of dementia', gives a good explanation of all the ways of looking at dementia and explaining it, alongside details of the variations and the possible risk factors.

Holden, U. and Stokes, G. (2002) 'The "Dementias".' In G. Stokes and F. Goudie (eds), *The Essential Dementia Care Handbook*. Bicester: Speechmark.

This is an excellent book and this chapter (Chapter 2) gives a good overview of the various forms of dementia.

Stokes, G. and Goudie, E. (1990) *Working with Dementia*. Bicester: Winslow Press.

Chapter 2

History of Dementia and Dementia Care

Key message
Over 20 per cent of the over-80s will suffer some form of dementia and most dementia sufferers are being cared for in the community by their families.

The word 'dementia' has been around for quite some time and comes from the Latin *demens* which literally means 'without mind'. The Greeks, including Plato, recognised it as an abnormal condition of old age. By the eighteenth century it was becoming medically recognised as 'abolition of the reasoning faculty', according to a French scientific encyclopaedia of 1765 (Berrios 1994). However, it was not until the mid-nineteenth century that dementia of early onset became recognised as a specific medical entity. It was then associated with cognitive impairment, memory decline and a decline in social functioning.

For many the workhouse was the only care option until the Victorians built the large asylums. In 1907 Dr Alois Alzheimer published a paper identifying a cluster of symptoms of dementia. These included reduced comprehension and memory, disorientation, unpredictable behaviour and difficulties with communication. Thus Alzheimer's disease was born. There was then a period of very little research into dementia and care for sufferers was largely ignored. If not cared for at home many dementia sufferers were cared for in long-stay 'psycho-geriatric' wards. With the decline of NHS long-term care in the 1980s, institutional care of dementia is now largely a function of private residential and nursing homes. The issue of responsibility for long-term care and dementia care generally has long been a bone of contention between health and social services. There is still much debate as to whether caring for a dementia sufferer is a nursing or a social task. In Scotland long-term care for dementia is free, as it is seen as a nursing task. However, in the rest of the UK politicians regard the care as being primarily social in nature.

In the 1970s pre-senile dementia such as Alzheimer's was largely regarded as untreatable and was rarely acted upon or brought to the attention of specialist services, of which there were few, and there had been very little research into the disease. Cheston and Bender (1999) point out that during the 1970s there was a

Discussion point

Discuss amongst your colleagues these contentious points:

- Is caring for a person with dementia a nursing or a social task?

- Is it both?

- At what stage might it change and why?

- Who should pay for such caring services, whether they are health or social in nature?

realisation that increases in life expectancy would result in greater numbers of dementia sufferers. In the UK in 1930 the average life expectancies were 59 years for men and 68 for women. By 1970 these had risen to 63 and 74. This had huge implications for health and social policy and it is because of the large numbers of people involved that the financing of such care is a contentious issue. The Alzheimer's Society estimate the prevalence figures for dementia in 2001 to be two per cent of the over-65s, five per cent of the over-70s and 20 per cent of the over-80s. The Health Advisory Service report *The Rising Tide* (1983) highlighted these demographic concerns with its title. At the same time there was a growing realisation that not only was dementia a major cause of ill health in later life, it was actually a major cause of death. Traditionally in many cases pneumonia or some other known illness has been given as the cause of death, as these were indeed the micro cause, but the reality is that it is the dementia that kills.

Since the 1980s the profile of dementia has been raised and how it is viewed has changed. Sufferers are no longer seen as unfortunate victims of diseased brains for whom little can be done, but as fellow human beings capable of responding and enjoying human relationships and having a full bill of rights. The model of care has also evolved from one of containment and pity to one of normalisation and inclusion. The emphasis is on improving sufferers' quality of life and making it as enjoyable as possible. This is difficult work and improving the quality of life of a dementia sufferer remains one of the greatest challenges facing the caring professions. But we have begun to recognise ways in which we can meaningfully interact with people with dementia in ways which can make a real difference to them. The formation of the Alzheimer's Disease Society in 1979 (now called the Alzheimer's Society) has also helped to raise the profile of dementia issues and to foster more positive approaches to care. The work of Tom Kitwood (Kitwood and Bredin 1991) in the 1980s and 1990s has also helped take dementia care forwards and away from a purely medical model. Kitwood's work gives us a more holistic view which puts social and psychological factors to the fore, emphasises helping the sufferer achieve personhood and focuses on retaining individuality.

Research into the biology of dementia has also provided a group of drugs called 'anti-cholinesterase inhibitors', which can temporarily delay the worst effects of the dementia for some people in the initial stages. But dementia remains untreatable in any real sense and it is improvements in caring which largely will have an impact upon improving a sufferer's quality of life.

With the bulk of sufferers being cared for at home in the community (roughly 80 per cent, according to the Alzheimer's Society) it is also important to have good community support and service provision. However, the truth is that it is somewhat of a lottery as to what is available in any one given area. There is enormous geographic variation. There has been a long legacy of government reports, white papers and research studies which tell us exactly what carer's needs are, but little money has followed through to make these provisions a reality. Many carers struggle to cope and the situation of caring has been termed the 'burden of care'. The *National Service Framework for Mental Health* (1999) focuses only upon working age adults and one has to look to the *National Service Framework for Older People* (Department of Health 2001) to find reference to dementia. This might be another example of the marginalisation of dementia which, given the scale of the problem, many argue would deserve a National Service Framework in its own right.

Further reading and references

Alzheimer's Society (2004) Alzheimer's Society policy position paper – *Demography*. Available at www.alzheimers.org.uk

Berrios, G. (1994) 'Dementia: historical overview.' In A. Burns and R. Levy (eds) *Dementia*. London: Chapman Hall.

Cheston, R. and Bender, M. (1999) *Understanding Dementia: The Man with the Worried Eyes*. London: Jessica Kingsley Publishers.
  Chapter 1 gives an interesting account of the history of dementia and the issues surrounding its medicalisation.

Department of Health (1999) *National Service Framework for Mental Health: London: The Stationery Office*.

Department of Health (2001) *National Service Framework for Older People*. London: DoH.

Health Advisory Service (1983) *The Rising Tide*. Sutton: HAS.

Kings Fund (1986) *Living Well into Old Age: Applying Principles of Good Practice to Services for Elderly People with Severe Mental Impairment*. London: Kings Fund.

Chapter 3

How Dementia Affects Us

Key message

Before embarking on a description of the common symptoms and typical progression of a dementia, it is important to remind ourselves that everybody will experience, present and progress through a dementia differently. Sufferers will share certain common trends and behaviours, but they will retain strong aspects of their own individuality. In bad practice scenarios everyone is treated alike, with a blanket application of standard care procedures because they all suffer from dementia. The focus of care should be unique and individual, not based on the dementia; it is easy to lose sight of the person behind the label. A dementia cannot eliminate the effects of so many variables; there will always be a high degree of uniqueness in any sufferer.

Miesen (1992) suggests that the experience of dementia can be understood and described as a sort of 'strange situation' which becomes more permanent. The more vague or strange the situation, the more people with dementia cling to what is familiar and what or who they can identify. These familiar faces and objects become an important source of reassurance but one that is gradually eroding with the sufferer's memory. It is difficult to feel exactly what it must be like to suffer from dementia, but it is possible to empathise with just how frightening and frustrating this sort of sensation and strangeness must be.

Others have suggested it is like being placed on a strange planet where you cannot understand the language or behaviour of the other beings, who are constantly doing to you things you can't understand. There is no one you can turn to for clarification or help. You are trapped in a totally unfathomable world. Nothing makes any sense whatsoever. You try to make sense of things and all you get is bisd Shdfu perinff fugfn mjchfifm jjdhjd; pwvr ndophjsdfe bdgdg.

Common symptoms

Memory and disorientation

Short-term memory is affected in dementia and typically in the mid- to latter stages the client can remember little of what has recently happened but can recall events from the distant past. In the early stages of the dementia sufferers often have insight into their failing memory and failing cognitive ability and this leads them to confabulate or make up stories to cover their mistakes or memory lapses. Errors, lapses and mistakes start to affect their work performance and home life and they may attempt to cover these up, sometimes doing this so well that it is hard for even those close to them to pick up on them. This is part of the reason that dementia is often not detected until it is well advanced. Such confabulations are of course a protective mechanism or a method of denial by the sufferer. It is obviously very frightening to realise that you are losing your mind.

> **Discussion point**
>
> Gladys is wandering up and down the main corridor trying all the doors and occasionally stopping to stare out of the window. She looks frightened and turns away from those who approach her, shouting, 'What?', 'What?'.
>
> What would you do about this?

Later on, as the dementia progresses, the person can find it hard to remember what it is they are supposed to be doing, or where they are. How to perform simple tasks such as dressing can be forgotten.

> **Discussion point**
>
> Gladys sits on the side of the bed struggling with a skirt, which she keeps wrapping around one of her legs. Eventually she gives up, gets up and wanders around the room.
>
> What would you do about this?
>
> What about tomorrow?

Sufferers will also find it hard to remember who other people are and it is particularly hard for close relatives and friends to realise that they are no longer recognised.

Often it can seem as if the client is living in the past, as indeed they are: if what is in their minds is a memory from a long time ago, then that is the reality for them. Sufferers may also be disorientated about time, becoming increasingly confused as to what time of day it is; they may for instance get up in the middle of the night believing it is the morning.

Cognitive ability

The decline in intellectual ability makes it difficult for the sufferer to make sense of the world around them. Their ability to process information erodes; they cannot work things out or make sense of what is going on around them and cannot learn new things. Their vocabulary declines and communication becomes impaired as their ability to recognise what is said diminishes, alongside the ability to form their own speech. They cannot name objects or explain. They thus become increasingly cut off from a world they can't understand or communicate with. Compounding this is a reduction in their concentration span; the sufferer will be slow to respond. They may repeat phrases as if they are somehow trying to make sense of them. Ultimately many sufferers will speak in what to us are jumbles of meaningless words.

Mood

Changes of mood can be a common feature, with depression, irritability and frustration all being understandable responses to the sufferer's situation and inability to make sense of what's going on around them.

Behaviour

There are many behaviours which, if seen in the context of the sufferer's disintegrating and frightening world, are entirely understandable. Yet because we find them hard to cope with we often label them as 'difficult behaviours'. Most of these are born of fear and frustration. Imagine not realising where you are. Then two strangers suddenly come up to you and start trying to take off your clothes. You resist and they try harder, they are speaking in riddles and forcing you towards a strange white contraption. A realistic response to such a scenario would almost inevitably get you labelled as aggressive. Yet aggression in self-defence would be an entirely appropriate response. Declining abilities to perform the activities of daily living mean that there are many such times when sufferers must suffer interventions they do not understand. The list of what to us might seem like inappropriate behaviours also includes wandering, disinhibition, difficulties with eating, dressing and personal hygiene, toileting problems, repetition, accusations, screaming and withdrawal.

Personality

The stress of the dementia may also bring forth changes in personality so that a once quiet and mild-mannered gentleman may become uncharacteristically aggressive and argumentative. Similarly, a previously confident and domineering woman may withdraw into herself. Such drastic personality changes are hard for close family members to come to terms with.

Progression

Three stages of dementia have traditionally been identified and a crude form of classification such as this can help to gauge the rate of progress of the illness. The stages are based on the progression of Alzheimer's disease.

- *Mild dementia* – There can be an unwillingness to try out new things or ideas and an inability to adapt to change. It becomes difficult to retain new information. Tell-tale signs of memory loss such as repeating oneself or forgetfulness and misplacing things become apparent. There might be a tendency to blame others for mishaps or make excuses for memory lapses. Routines are clung to amidst a growing fear of the unfamiliar. Withdrawal is a common feature and can be seen as an attempt to avoid failure. Often the signs are taken to be part of the normal ageing process or put down to stress. The sufferer may begin to lose interest in their hobbies, work and socialising. They may find it hard to concentrate and make decisions. There may also be a degree of insight which could show itself as depression, fear or frustration. It is a time during which a great deal of support and reassurance is required.

- *Moderate dementia* – Long-term memory comes to the fore as short-term memory is severely reduced. More and more things will become cloudy and uncertain. The sufferer believes they are living in the past recreated by their long-term memories. Disorientation becomes more apparent with sufferers doing things at inappropriate times of the day: going to bed before lunch and getting up in the middle of the night are common examples. With increasing forgetfulness the sufferer may begin to forget names and lose recognition of close friends and family. This forgetting and losing of things can lead to much frustration. Repetition of questions increases. Wandering becomes a frequent occurrence as sufferers lose recognition of their surroundings. Deteriorating personal hygiene becomes more apparent. More and more help is needed with everyday tasks such as dressing and eating. There is a greater element of risk at this stage as sufferers may forget to light the gas on their cooker, leave the door to their home open or get lost. The growing confusion can also begin to manifest itself in behaviours such as inappropriate dressing or toileting. There is increasing social withdrawal, frustration and depression. There can also be inappropriate or disinhibited behaviour. Language skills will deteriorate to the stage whereby communication becomes very difficult.

- *Severe dementia* – At this stage sufferers cannot understand speech or communicate by it. Memory is almost completely lost. Sufferers can often become very disturbed as they search for meaning. The world becomes an unrecognisable place which the sufferer may wish to withdraw from or rebel against. Wandering and general restlessness increases and they cannot undertake simple activities of daily living such as feeding and dressing. To them, the help given by carers must feel like an army of strange people are interfering with them. However, even at this late stage they are still able to respond to affection and benefit from caring relationships. Eventually they experience physical changes such as weight loss, incontinence and general frailty. The sufferer will often come to need 24-hour nursing care and for many the end is a bedridden, immobile state. Often an illness such as a chest infection or pneumonia is the ultimate cause of death.

Further reading and references

Forsythe, E. (1990) *Alzheimer's Disease: The Long Bereavement*. London: Faber.

Goldsmith, M. (1996) 'Different people are affected in different ways.' In M. Goldsmith, *Hearing the Voice of People with Dementia: Opportunities and Obstacles*. London: Jessica Kingsley Publishers.

In this chapter Goldsmith makes a plea for us not to 'lump' all the different dementias together but to regard them as separate because they will have different effects upon people. Dementia sufferers are very different people being affected by different illnesses. This means that there will be a need for individual care and not just the blanket application of standard 'dementia care'. Goldsmith also points out that social and psychological factors influence the symptoms someone gets and the way the illness progresses. So you now have different people, different illnesses and different social and psychological factors which all ensure that no two dementia presentations are the same, each needing a unique, individualised care package.

Kitwood, T. and Bredin, K. (1991) *Person to Person: A Guide to the Care of Those with Failing Mental Powers*. Second edition. Loughton: Gale Publications.

Miesen, B. (1992) 'Attachment theory and dementia'. In G. Jones and B. Miesen (eds) *Care Giving in Dementia*. London: Routledge.

Exercise 3.1

FACTORS THAT MAKE PEOPLE DIFFERENT

Think individually about what it is that makes us different from each other. Jot down your ideas below and then discuss your lists with your group.

The following are some of the factors: genetics, biology, brain structure, education, upbringing and childhood, social background, ethnicity, gender, religion, temperament, personality, introvert/extrovert, health, coping skills, finances, poverty, culture, lifestyle, hobbies, values, beliefs, family ties, marriage, work history, relationships, friends, personal tastes (food, clothes etc.), politics, travel, art, sport, sex, diet, personal care, where you lived, life experiences.

Exercise 3.2

INSIGHT INTO HOW IT FEELS TO HAVE DEMENTIA

Given the descriptions above of how dementia progresses and affects us, draw up a list with your colleagues of what might be going through the mind of a sufferer in the early stages who has retained some insight into their condition.

- What might their emotions, feelings and thoughts be?

- How might you help here?

Exercise 3.3

THE IMPORTANCE OF SUPPORT

You are losing your sense of reality and finding it hard to keep in touch with what is going on around you. You are becoming increasingly unaware of what and where this place is; the surroundings seem more and more unfamiliar. You occasionally find yourself in places you do not recognise and are not sure how to get home or where home is. You are not sure what you should be doing and find it hard to understand what people are saying or who they are. Things seem to make less sense these days. You seem not to be able to do anything or understand much about your situation: it is all very hazy. Lots of strangers somehow begin to feature in your life.

In the early stages of dementia you retain some insight into the fact that all is not well. This must be a nightmare scenario which is difficult for most of us to envisage, but we can try and understand just how frightening and humiliating such an existence might be. Imagine then the importance of the understanding and support of those around you.

- What do you think is important here in terms of support?

- How will we demonstrate that support and understanding?

- Brain storm a list of ways we can do this?

- Think about the ways in which a client with dementia might find it hard to recognise or understand this support.

Chapter 4

Attitudes and Needs

Key message

The attitude we hold about people tends to colour the way we interact with them. Much of the bad practice that we witness at times stems directly from a negative attitude towards those with dementia.

There is undoubtedly still a large degree of ageism in society generally. Old age is viewed by many as a slow decline into decay and boredom alongside increasing physical and mental frailty. Older people are viewed as stubborn, slow and burdensome. They drive too slowly, they amble along dragging their shopping trolleys behind them, getting under everyone's feet. There are always lots of them in the supermarket queue slowing things down and then only buying two things. These are all common perceptions and grumbles you will be familiar with. Yet they are all stereotypes arising from faulty thinking. We simply do not register and remember older people who do not fit this stereotype because we don't notice them. Like much else in life we have a tendency to remember the negative. It is similar to the way we give opinions: we are quick to complain but rarely give compliments. Most businesses have a complaints procedure; few have a compliments procedure!

Working in the caring professions can give you a skewed view of old age and it can be easy to slip into a mode of thinking in which all old people are physically and mentally frail and have little social life. However, this simply is not the case. Most older people are getting on with their lives quite happily, as Exercise 4.7 (pp.34–5) shows.

The single most important aspect of caring is our attitude towards our clients. There is a good way and a bad way of doing everything. In caring for the confused there is no perfect way of doing things, but our attitude to our clients will determine the quality of care we give them.

If we see our clients as awkward, slow, dementing and problematic, our care will be uncaring. If, however, we see them as unique individuals striving to come to terms with declining abilities, if we can see their history and find the person beyond the confusion, then our care will be caring.

We have a choice. We can see the ex-footballer, the father and husband who loved camping and who lived for his children and his dog, or we can see the incontinent old man who spills his tea and is troublesome about being toileted.

Attitudes are a powerful force and they will colour all we do, and clients can sense the care or carelessness in our approach. A negative attitude will give the client a sense of uselessness and of being rejected if we hurry them, a feeling of worthlessness if we ignore them, but a positive attitude will give them warmth, respect and the feeling of being valued as a person.

The easiest way of doing this is to always ask the question: 'How would I like to be treated?'

'Dementiaism'

Older people are discriminated against, but older people with mental health problems, especially dementia, carry a double burden. The biological model of dementia has been accused of leading to the depersonalisation of dementia sufferers. The model seems to suggest that sufferers are not alert, that they cannot be aware and have no real sense of self. This is tantamount to saying that the person no longer exists and that there is just a body with dementia. This is an extreme view, but all too often people focus not on the person but on the illness. They lose sight of the individual and are left with just a series of what are regarded as difficult-to-deal-with behaviours. Care becomes just a need to keep people clean, fed and watered, because it is felt that they can't appreciate anything beyond this. It is almost as if they have no worth. Examining such an extreme and negative view is valuable because it reminds us of what is important, namely respect for human dignity and individuality in our care. If we can see beyond the disease we can avoid such 'dementiaist' attitudes. All dementia sufferers are different not the same. Of course, caring for those with dementia would be simpler if you regarded everybody as the same, or as objects. Indeed this is how abuse creeps in. But if you recognise individual potentials, life histories and differences, the caring task becomes much more complex and interesting. Instead of regarding behaviour as difficult we can come to see behaviour as having real meaning for each individual, and then we might begin to try and interpret that behaviour and look for the meaning instead of merely regarding it as hard to deal with. Why is the person wandering? Why is the person screaming? Why is the person banging on the window or refusing their food? Such a search for meaning in otherwise apparently meaningless behaviour is an attempt to search for the person behind the behaviour. It is an attempt to focus on personhood rather than illness.

Institutional 'dementiaism' can be seen in many ways. Often dementia is seen as a natural part of ageing and GPs often do not refer sufferers on to specialist services – these can be perceived as forms of institutional 'dementiaism'. Since the behaviours exhibited in dementia, the ones we find difficult to deal with, are stigmatising, they often exclude sufferers from nursing home or residential placements and, more often, community-based facilities including day care. Such behaviours can also stigmatise the carers of those being cared for at home: carers may be seen as not coping or not looking after their loved ones properly. For professionals, the speciality of dementia care is often considered the least popular option rather than the highly skilled and rewarding challenge that it is.

Research

Research perhaps is affected by another subtle aspect of 'dementiaism'. Goldsmith (1999) points out that in 1996 in the UK £10 per sufferer was spent on dementia research, while £15,000 was spent per sufferer on AIDS research. At the time the numbers of sufferers were about 750,000 for dementia and 12,000 for AIDS!

Disability Discrimination Act 1995

This Act makes it unlawful to discriminate on the basis of disability and it offers legal protection to people with dementia. Visit the website www.disability.gov.uk/dda in order to explore this more.

Discussion point

How might the Disability Discrimination Act be used to protect the rights of your clients?

Treating people with dementia less favourably than others is now illegal. Our clients have the same rights to services, goods and facilities as others and should not be excluded from any activity or place on grounds of their dementia.

Health and Social Care National Occupational Standards

This chapter relates to many of the induction and foundation standards but in particular to the following level standards:

Level 2 core units

HSC21b Listen to and respond to individuals' questions and concerns.
HSC23a Evaluate your work.
HSC24b Treat people with respect and dignity.

Level 2 optional units

HSC234 a + b Ensure your own actions support the equality, diversity, rights and responsibilities of individuals.

Level 3 core units

HSC33 a + b Reflect on and develop your practice.

HSC 35 a, b + c Promote choice, well-being and the protection of all individuals.

Level 3 optional units

HSC3111 a + b Promote equality, diversity rights and responsibilities of individuals.

Level 4 core units

HSC43 a + b Take responsibility for the continuing professional development of self and others.

Mental Health Standards

D4.1 Identify individuals' needs and circumstances.

Care Homes for Older People: National Minimum Standards

10.5 Treat people with respect at all times.

32.1 The registered manager ensures that the management approach of the home creates an open, positive and inclusive atmosphere.

Further reading and references

Goldsmith, M. (1999) 'Ethical dilemmas in dementia care.' In T. Adams and C. Clarke (eds), *Dementia Care: Developing Partnerships in Practice*. London: Bailliere Tindall.

Kingston, P. (1999) *Ageism in History*. Nursing Times Clinical Monograph No 28. London: Emap Healthcare Ltd.

This is an extremely good summary of aspects of ageism throughout history. It also looks at contemporary issues, the role of the media, health care rationing and elder abuse.

New, B. and LeGrand, J. (1996) *Rationing in the National Health Service: Principles and Pragmatism*. London: King's Fund.

WHO (World Health Organisation) (2002) *Reducing Stigma and Discrimination Against Older People with Mental Disorders*. Geneva: WHO. Available at www.who.int

Exercise 4.1

STEREOTYPES

- Brain storm a list of negative stereotypes of older people.

- Discuss the truth of each one you come up with and where the stereotype might come from.

Exercise 4.2

ATTITUDES TO DEMENTIA

Think now about those with dementia. With your colleagues brain storm a list of commonly held attitudes and negative images you have come across. Write them down on a flip chart. Examine each one to discover if it is really true and try to come up with a counter-argument. Are we talking about everyone with dementia or just many different individuals with many different presentations?

Are the following true or false?

- The majority of the over-80s have dementia.

- The majority of dementia sufferers live in institutions.

- All people with dementia wander.

- All people with dementia are aggressive.

✔

Exercise 4.3

HOW DO WE SEE OUR CLIENTS?

This exercise examines how we could see our clients. The awkward old man might have been a keen runner, the slow eater a devoted father, the confused woman a dog lover, the incontinent woman a marvellous gardener. The restless wanderer is also a husband, the problematic client was a happy chap, the client with severe dementia was a headteacher and the rather messy eater devoutly religious.

There is a choice in how we see people. We can focus on the here-and-now difficulties they present to us as carers or we can look beyond this to find the person underneath.

- Identify how each of your clients might be regarded in a negative way because of some aspect of their behaviour.

- Then list a positive quality of their life which could make people regard them differently.

- In a staff group write a list of members' names and then list their positive qualities.

- Which aspects of their own lives would group members wish future carers to focus upon?

Exercise 4.4

STIGMA

Stigma results from a process whereby certain individuals and groups are unjustifiably rendered shameful, are excluded and discriminated against (WHO 2002). I can recall, during my nurse training, a day when clients with dementia were excluded from a trip to the seaside because of the possibility of their being incontinent. This was an example of the effects of stigma.

- Why was it unfair?

- How does such discrimination have a negative impact?

- How could any perceived difficulties have been overcome?

Exercise 4.5

DISCRIMINATION

'Discrimination' means any distinction, exclusion or preference that has the effect of nullifying or impairing equal enjoyment of rights (WHO 2002).

Can you think of any ways in which discrimination operates within your working environment and care home?

Exercise 4.6

AGEISM

'Ageism' is basically stereotyping and discrimination purely and simply because people are old. It is as bad as racism and sexism and has no place in modern society. Yet it is subtle and many people do not regard it as equally serious to the other 'ism's.

The media, for example, get away with ageist images of bumbling forgetfulness and oddity; if they did the same for race and gender they would find themselves in court. One often only sees older people in advertisements for laxatives, vitamins and insurance or as quirky individuals in soap operas. Positive use of the media showing older people in leadership roles and as popular figures can go a long way to overcoming ageist stereotypes, but such portrayals are rare.

There is also a sort of 'institutionalised' ageism, an acceptance of discrimination against older people. There is evidence that upon reaching a certain age access to health care starts to get rationed (New and LeGrand 1996). An older person might get an obligatory check-up from their GP, but they may not get access to all treatments. The evidence suggests that older people are denied treatment not because it will not work but because it is not seen as cost effective. It is almost as if the severity of illness declines with age. Such negative attitudes are an expression of the belief that older people are not worth helping and as a result they are often denied treatment for improvable physical and psychological ills.

Even if an older adult is not severely ill but in need of care there is a subtle implication of lack of importance. Why can you earn more money stacking the shelves or working the tills of a supermarket than you can by providing care for older people?

Discuss the implications of this.

The great bulk of institutional care for older people is entrusted to unqualified personnel and such work is often regarded as unskilled. Yet to do it properly requires enormous amounts of skill and patience. Throw dementia into the equation and the skills required of care workers become huge.

✓

Exercise 4.7

TRUE OR FALSE?

Answer true or false to each question.

1. Intelligence declines with age.

2. Most older people have no interest in sex.

3. Most older people live alone.

4. Most older people are set in their ways and resistant to change.

5. Most older people are alike.

6. Most older people are bored.

7. Most older people are socially isolated and lonely.

8. Forty per cent of the population of the UK are over-65.

9. Most older people are grumpy and depressed.

10. The majority of the over-80s have dementia.

11. The majority of dementia sufferers live in institutions.

12. All people with dementia wander.

13. All people with dementia are aggressive.

The answers to this exercise can be found on the next page.

Dementia Care Training Manual for Staff Working in Nursing and Residential Settings © Danny Walsh 2006

ANSWERS TO EXERCISE 4.7

1. False. Older people usually achieve the same IQ scores, though it might take them a bit longer to do the test.

2. False. Most older people remain sexually active.

3. False. Only women in the over-75 age range are more likely to live alone and this is largely because men tend to die at a younger age.

4. False. This is a common stereotype. Older people have to adapt to many changes and many younger people are set in their ways.

5. False. There is as much variation amongst the older generation as there is in other generations.

6. False. Most are actively engaged or have good social networks.

7. False. Even with the decline of the extended family and greater social mobility most older adults are still visited by relatives who live close by.

8. False. The 2002 statistics put it at 18.4 per cent.

9. False. There are high suicide rates among older adults but the overwhelming majority enjoy their lives.

10. False. Only about 20 per cent have dementia.

11. False. Only about 20 per cent are in institutions, the majority being cared for in their own homes.

12. False. Wandering is a common symptom but by no means universal.

13. False. This is a common stereotype and while it may be a feature of some presentations it is by no means universal or inevitable. Most aggression in dementia arises from poor care.

Chapter 5

Communication in Dementia

Key messages

- All communication has meaning no matter how nonsensical to us.
- There is always a hidden message that we need to get in touch with.
- Focus on feelings.

Good, clear communication skills are essential in dementia care because we know that confusion has profound effects on a sufferer's ability to communicate. In the early stages of dementia it can often take some time for sufferers to make sense of what is said or to find the words they want to say. Later on they may not be able to understand what is said to them or make responses, and in the even later stages of dementia they may only utter what to us are meaningless jumbles of sounds. Because of these factors it is important to bear in mind some basic principles.

> **Discussion point**
> The saying 'silent care is bad care' is particularly true in dementia. Why is this so?

All communication has meaning

A basic principle to bear in mind is that all messages and communications have meaning, no matter how nonsensical they might seem to us. They have a meaning for the sufferer and it is up to us to try and work it out or second guess it. This underlines the importance of knowing your clients as individuals and becoming familiar with their communication patterns and idiosyncrasies. Once you achieve such familiarity you will understand more. One client, for example, would begin to walk in a tight circle whenever he wanted the toilet; similarly it was possible to recognise the meaning behind some of his strange words once the time was taken to look for patterns and listen. It is very important to remember the importance of non-verbal communication in dementia, so look for the non-verbal clues. Facial expressions and body language can convey much about how people feel and act as a window into the client's emotional state. Remember that the sufferer will be reading your body language and facial expressions. So be calm in your approach as agitation or frustration on your part will be recognised and this will be upsetting. The perception of confidence will be reassuring for the sufferer.

Focus on feelings

As well as meanings, all messages have a 'feeling' component and it is crucial to remember this. The ability of dementia sufferers to feel and express emotions remains intact. Because of this we know that the emotions they express are those which are being felt. This allows us to validate the client's emotions and share happiness or comfort in sadness. Thus, if we can no longer recognise the sufferer's words we should try to guess, and if we can't do that we should focus on the feelings being displayed. Try to reflect in your own facial expressions the emotional state of the sufferer, so that they can try and pick up the message that you understand how they feel. Laugh and smile or look sad when appropriate.

Common communication problems

Dysphasia

Dysphasia can be receptive dysphasia, which is an inability to understand the meaning of words, or expressive dysphasia, the inability to produce speech. Typically, people with dysphasia might just say 'dink' to indicate that they want a drink. The sound uttered may not be a recognisable word but, by paying attention to patterns, it is possible to recognise what someone is trying to say. An in-depth knowledge of the individual will allow you to imagine what they want and you can check it out by asking questions which only need a yes or no answer or a nod.

Repetition

This often takes the form of the sufferer repeating the same question over and over again as they have forgotten that they have asked it. Responses and other phrases can also be repeated, even the same word or sound. It can be a sign of distress, so try and guess the cause of any anxiety. However, it may be a source of comfort, a bit like repeating or chanting a mantra.

Slowness

Slowness is seen most often in the rate of giving a response. When dementia starts to exert an effect upon the ability to communicate and understand language it might take some time for the sufferer to get to grips with what is being said. Sufferers may need to mull over in their heads what is being said to them and think about it before they fully understand. They then must also take some time to sort out what it is they wish to say in return and how to say it. Giving the person the time to understand, repeating the question if necessary and allowing them time to form their response will help them to succeed in communicating. The bad practice scenario is not taking time and rushing on; this in effect cuts off the opportunity for the client to communicate. We are back to a golden rule: you cannot rush dementia care.

Talking continually

It can be very irritating for carers when people with dementia talk continuously, especially if what they say is nonsensical to us. As with repetition, it may be either a sign of distress or a source of comfort. Seek out any obvious cause of anxiety. If none is apparent then so be it: tolerate the continuous talking or try to engage with it. Often the cause of such communication is a desire to be recognised and for company.

Non-communication

Non-communication can be a major problem for carers: it can be soul destroying for a loved one to withdraw into a world where they only communicate if you initiate it. This is not apathy and they are not being indifferent, they have merely lost the skill of initiating conversation. If a person has lost some ability to understand language then it will be increasingly difficult for them to actually start a conversation. What is required here is that you initiate the conversation and provide the opportunity to communicate. In a busy care schedule and working day this need not be too time consuming. Short bursts of interaction and communication throughout the day can be worked into most schedules. Make this a priority. Care without communication becomes merely hotel care: the meals and the décor are nice, but clients are unstimulated.

Losing track

Often clients will lose the thread of what they were saying and regain it, sometimes with an entirely unrelated point. This is a result of their diminishing ability to both concentrate and understand the language they are trying to use. Gently remind the person of what they were saying and the point they were making. Take up the conversation for them if necessary, bringing them back to where they were.

Meaningless jumbles of letters and words

In the latter stages of dementia the sufferer will have lost the ability to understand and use language completely and will communicate in ways which we find hard to understand. We will not be able to understand the strange and seemingly meaningless utterances we hear. It is now that we need to use a validation therapy approach and remember that all communication, no matter how non-sensical, has meaning and feelings attached. So try and second-guess the meaning of what is being communicated and respond appropriately to the feelings being expressed. Laugh alongside happiness and comfort distress.

Naming difficulties

This is a frequent problem which can appear in the early stages of dementia. People will get the name of something or someone wrong, struggle to remember what it is called or use the wrong word. A gentle reminder or prompt will usually help as it is often clear what was meant. It can be especially hard for a carer when the sufferer can no longer remember their name. Think about this in the context of your own life and your loved ones and it is easy to feel how heartbreaking this must be. The memory loss causing this can also mean the sufferer might also make mistakes with people's roles. Husbands can become sons or fathers, sisters might be responded to as mothers. Again, this must be hard to bear.

Good communication

- *Communication aids* – Ensure that glasses are clean and that hearing aids are working properly. Such things are easily overlooked and it is easy to mistake confusion for a blocked hearing aid or flat batteries!

- *Environment* – It is important to keep background noise to a minimum when trying to talk, so turn televisions and music off or move to a quiet area. Clients often find it hard to concentrate and understand without having these other distractions.

- *Get attention* – Stop what you are doing. Do not try talking while you are doing something else, like making a bed, give all your attention to communicating. Before you start, make sure that you have got the person's attention. Get down to their level. Touch their arm to signal that you are going to speak, face them, get close, get eye contact and say their name.

- *Pace* – It is important not to rush, so speak slowly to allow people time to understand. Having said something, pause a while to give them time to make sense of what you have said and give them time to find the right words to respond. Check for understanding and if they look puzzled repeat what you said.

- *Tone* – Try to speak clearly and calmly without any signs of agitation or frustration. Sufferers will recognise the anger behind a raised voice.

- *Quantity/time* – Another important point is not to give several messages one after the other. Give one piece of information at a time and break this down into smaller parts if you need to. By doing this you are allowing time for people to understand. It will take them longer to process your words, so allow them the time and do not rush them. Use short sentences and stress key words. Multiple messages such as: 'Brenda, it's morning, time to get up, you need to get dressed, how about your blue jumper, it's poached eggs today and I think Sheila is coming', give the person little chance to either understand or respond and can heighten their sense of loss and inability.

- *Be specific* – Try to use names of things and people, instead of using words such as 'he' or 'she'.

- *Non-verbals* – When verbal communication is diminished, non-verbal clues help enormously. A smile signifies much that words cannot and clients will recognise emotions and facial expressions long after the ability to recognise words is lost. So emphasise your facial expressions, give eye contact, use touch, gestures and pointing, mime simple tasks. The words 'Do you want to brush your teeth?' may be meaningless but your mime may trigger the memory of what you are asking. Use nods, 'uh huhs', and 'mmms' to show that you are listening and to maintain the interaction.

- *Touch* – Touch is important because it is reassuring and also useful in gaining attention. A squeeze of the hand can help to maintain a conversation as well as giving the message you care for the person. Just holding hands or massaging the hands will help to reiterate the message that they are valued.

- *Practice* – When we know that communication skills are declining for our clients we should try to provide the opportunity for practising and maintaining them by spending time with the person for no other purpose than this. Look at a magazine together, spend 15 minutes in the garden – many opportunities exist which can provide a useful short and meaningful interaction. You need to consciously set aside time to do this: it is easily overlooked. Clients who are in the later stages of dementia often can't initiate interaction and have little language ability left. Use such times to focus on feelings and use non-verbal methods such as touch, alongside praise and encouragement, to communicate your appreciation of their company.

Avoid

Avoid asking direct and open questions if you can, because this can lead to feelings of frustration if the sufferer cannot come up with the response. If you need to use questions try and use those which only need a yes or no answer. It can be confusing to have to make choices so offer the answer – for example, ask 'Shall we have a cup of tea?' rather than 'What would you like to drink?'

Be there

Even if the two of you cannot understand each other and there are lengthy silences, do not give up. Stay with the client and show that you are still there for them. Use touch, hold hands, have a cuddle, do whatever is appropriate for that individual sufferer, perhaps just sit together for a while. By not abandoning them you are giving them the powerful message that even in the face of not being able to understand each other you still value them and want to be with them.

Health and Social Care National Occupational Standards

This chapter relates to many of the induction and foundation standards but in particular to the following level standards:

Level 2 core units

HSC 21 a, b + c Communicate with and complete records for individuals.

Level 3 core units

HSC31 a, b + c Promote effective communication for and about individuals.

Level 3 optional units

HSC369 a, b + c Support individuals with specific communication needs.

Mental Health Standards

A4.1 + 4.2 Promote effective communication and relationships.
A6.1, 6.2, 6.3 Promote effective communication where there are communication differences.
G1.1, 1.2, 1.3 Establish, sustain and disengage from relationships with clients.

Further reading and references

Norberg, A. (1999) 'Communication with people suffering with severe dementia.' In M. Clinton and S. Nelson (eds) *Advanced Practice in Mental Health Nursing.* Oxford: Blackwell Science.

Chapter 6

Individualised Care and Client History

Key messages

- Each person with dementia is unique.
- Dementia affects us all differently.
- Care should be individualised.
- The more you know about the client, the better the care will be.

There are several forms of dementia and over 750,000 individual variations of it currently in the UK. Dementia, no matter what the type, affects us all differently because we are all different. Even if you can identify the type of dementia, remember that all people do not get it to the same degree and that there is not just one form that affects us all the same way. We also all have unique histories, coping skills and personalities as well as many other individual facets, and therefore we will react differently to the onset and experience of the symptoms of dementia. Our brains are unique, having different abilities and biological variation. Thus, since there are different variations of dementia affecting thousands of personalities that are each unique, there can be no one way of coping. What we need to know in any one case is how this form of dementia affects this particular individual.

There will also be other factors affecting the way we are, such as physical health. In old age the senses may decline and this can give rise to communication difficulties. Some people are better in the mornings and some are slow starters but perk up as the day goes on. Similarly the environment has a huge impact upon us. However, for those clients in residential or nursing home settings, the single most important factor in alleviating some of the distress that dementia can bring is the quality of care received. The quality of that care will be much enhanced if it is tailored to each client's unique set of circumstances, history, personality and needs.

So, one of the most important ways of improving the quality of life of dementia sufferers is by embracing an individualised approach to care. It is bad practice to treat all clients alike despite their having differing needs. It is easy to see how clients are adjusted to the needs of the routine or institution rather than the other way around. Instead of applying the same care to everybody we should be adapting our approach to the particular needs of each individual client. Our clients might all have dementia, but underneath this label is a unique individual with a unique history and unique current needs. It is the task of carers to find the person beneath the label and get to know their clients well in order that they can tailor their care to their specific needs, preferences, values and habits.

Even when someone has severe dementia it is important that you seek the individual. While dementia can alter a client's personality to a degree, it cannot alter their past. Even the most severely demented client will retain a sense of individuality. As previously stated, we are all individuals and if we have dementia we will all dement in slightly different ways. We will not all merge into a oneness of dementia. Unless, that is, poor care succeeds in eroding the individuality we do retain.

Routine and individuality

It is often easier to see what to do for best by identifying what not to do. If we eradicate poor care then we are left with only good care. This is a simple truth but often it can be hard to see the wood for the trees. Sometimes we do things out of routine and without really thinking about what we are doing or why. Often we do things we feel are good but when we analyse them we can see how they might be done differently. So it is important to sit back sometimes and take a good look at what we are doing.

Good individualised care can combat some of the effects of dementia. Sometimes we pre-judge and make assumptions about a person because of the label 'dementia'. However, when we get to know the person underneath we can be pleasantly surprised. Tom Kitwood (1997a) illustrates how what he calls 'personhood' can be all too easily undermined. He cites examples of bad practice that ultimately lead to deterioration and a miserable existence for the sufferer. This will be explored in more detail in Chapter 12 on bad practice, but it is important here to argue that good practice can overcome this and one of the most important aspects of good practice is to get to know the clients as individuals very thoroughly.

Every one of us has a routine we like to stick to: it is a comfort and we can get upset if it is disturbed. In dementia this routine becomes especially important as it allows us to hang on to what is familiar when other things around us might be becoming unclear and confusing. It is easy to see then that, in an institutional setting, an individual's normal routines might be replaced by the institution's own.

Most of us, for example, will have a regular night-time routine in relation to the time we go to bed, what we like to have for supper, when we wash, when and how we brush our teeth, and what we do with our clothes. Maybe we check all the doors and feed the hamster. It is all very personal. This routine can be a source of great comfort and helps put us at ease, ready for sleep. Indeed, changes to that routine can lead to disturbed sleep. The obvious question arises then, in relation to our clients: what were their routines and how can we help them to adhere to them? Maybe it's the large scotch or two at the end of the day, maybe it's not retiring until after watching the news, maybe it's having a bath just after seven o'clock and sitting around in their dressing gown for a few hours. Your task is to get to know what it is or was for your clients and try to reinstate it if possible (see Exercises 6.2, 6.3 and 6.4, pp.49–50).

Choices, rights, options and strengths

Having choices in life is something we all take for granted but is often unwittingly eroded when we enter a nursing home or residential care as clients. The ability to make choices determines how we feel about ourselves in relation to self-esteem. If we are not able to make such decisions we can come to feel powerless and useless. It is important that we empower our clients in this area by providing them with the opportunity to make choices and decisions for themselves.

One way of delivering choices to clients is by making a list of their preferences, likes and dislikes. Only when armed with this information can you be prepared and offer that choice. You cannot offer someone coffee if you were not aware that they would prefer it and thus did not have any to offer. The simple act of finding out about a preference for a particular type of biscuit can make a huge difference to a client. Choices can be made in many areas, as Exercise 6.6 (p.51) will show.

When talking about choices and preferences it is pertinent to think about the effects of stereotyping. Knowing your client's individual preferences will help you to avoid falling into the trap of categorising them as belonging to any one stereotype. It is very easy to come to see older people as stereotypical of one generation or age group. The reality is that there is much variation. Not everybody likes popular music; there is much variation in musical taste. So when carers undertake reminiscence sessions about the 1940s they must not assume that all of the clients enjoyed the popular wartime songs such as 'Pack up your troubles'. Some may well have had a preference for jazz or classical music. It is important to bear these details in mind as they stop us blending everybody in together.

'Being with'

If we have a better understanding of our clients as individuals we will be better able to communicate with them, and in doing so our interactions will better meet their psychological needs and individual requirements. The more we recognise people as individuals, the better able we are to empathise with them and their predicament. Our attitude towards our clients will warm the better we get to know them.

It can be argued that once a cognitive decline has been recognised, stereotyping of dementia sufferers begins and many people reduce their interactions with sufferers. Communication becomes less frequent and expectations of the sufferer's abilities decline. With this scenario prevalent it is easy for sufferers to become increasingly isolated and neglected. This is a reaffirmation of their loss of individuality and worth and must do much to damage their already vulnerable self-esteem. What should happen, of course, is just the opposite. There should be more interaction and communication in order to combat the onset of cognitive decline. This will help the client retain a sense of self-worth and belonging.

Even in cases of severe dementia the client's uniqueness and identity will still remain. Getting in touch with this requires much communication and 'being with' but it will promote a degree of well-being not often expected in the face of such cognitive decline. Helping the client retain a sense of individuality can come down to just 'being with', by which we mean just spending time with the person to communicate to them they are worth spending time with and that we like being with them. Where verbal communication and understanding has been lost such simple humans skills can count for and mean a lot.

On a day-to-day basis, part of treating people in our care as individuals is about just spending time with them as individuals. Instead of rushing around doing things it is important to spend some time in one-to-one conversation with clients. It might not be long, and indeed a little and often might be the best or only possible way, but it will make a large difference to the client to know that you think they are worth the trouble of spending some time with.

Reminiscence

Reminiscence is a useful way of working with clients in order to expand our knowledge of them as individuals and for them to retain a sense of individuality. We will deal with it in depth in Chapter 9 but introduce here some useful one-to-one work you might undertake to foster individuality.

Personal scrapbook

This is an excellent excuse for much one-to-one work with a client. Buy a scrapbook and fill it with pictures of subjects relevant to your client's life and times. It might be possible to get old photographs of them at different stages of their life, for example at school, marriage, work etc. Put in pictures from areas they lived in, worked in or went on holiday to. Other aspects which can be covered are pets, hobbies, favourite sports teams and singers; the list is endless. See the individual profile section below and Chapter 9 for more pointers and ideas. The aim is that you then use this as an excuse for a chat and some individual time. It provides a focal point for a conversation which will also validate the client's sense of individuality.

Use the history and the individual profile in this chapter to help you build up a personal life history for each client. Think of it as building a sort of time line. The reminiscence section will give you good ideas for scrapbook items.

Personal history board

This presents another opportunity for stimulus, interaction and conversation, but again acts as a daily reminder for the client of their own individuality and uniqueness. Thus it is a valuable orientation aid. Basically you create a collage of personal photographs and mementos and it hangs in a prominent and easily viewed position, perhaps on a bedside locker or beside an armchair. You can do it in a large picture frame to make it look better. The opportunity will then be there to discuss it on a daily basis while helping people in the mornings or evenings or just spending some quiet time with them in their room.

The individual profile

The key to being able to deliver individualised care is in building up a thorough picture and history of the client. You can do this using many sources. Talking to the client is obviously the starting point and will give you a good basis upon which to build a good relationship. This should be a joint project, not something you are doing for the client but with them. Conversations with relatives and friends will help to fill in any gaps, as might any records you have. Only by this detailed individual history can you tailor your care to meet individual needs and begin to understand the uniqueness of the client in your care. Such a history will give you vital information regarding what made them 'tick', what they liked, valued and enjoyed, so that you can try to 're-provide' it.

In much the same way, you may be surprised about what you find out about your clients by getting a good history. It can radically alter your perceptions about them. The process can also be a good attitude changer. Goldsmith (1997) cites an American study in which care staff's impressions of clients' abilities were much greater for having read their life histories. The inside knowledge such a history gives you links the client to past achievements and abilities and therefore helps remove the low expectations that usually come with clients who have the label 'dementia'. A proforma entitled Individual Client Profile for taking a client's history and finding out those important individual details is provided on pp.55–58 (Exercise 6.11).

This is not supposed to be all-encompassing; in fact, we could go on expanding the categories the more we think about all the other aspects of life. However, this will give you a good basis to gain an understanding of your client's unique past life and current individual needs.

The next step is, of course, to fill in one of these for a client. Do it with the client and then ask relatives and friends to fill in the blanks with you. Check these out with the client. Once complete, sit down with your colleagues, relatives and the client, and try to come up with ways of individualising the care, given the client's history and passions.

Health and Social Care National Occupational Standards

This chapter relates to many of the induction and foundation standards but in particular to the following level standards:

Level 2 core units

HSC21b Listen to and respond to individuals' questions and concerns.
HSC24a Relate to and support individuals in the way they choose.

Level 2 optional units

HSC233 a + b Relate to and interact with individuals.
HSC234 a+ b Ensure your own actions support the equality, diversity, rights and responsibilities of individuals.

Level 3 core units

HSC33 a + b Reflect on and develop your practice.
HSC35 a + b Promote choice and independence and respect the diversity and difference of individuals.

Level 3 optional units

HSC332 a, b + c Support the social, emotional and identity needs of the individual.
HSC334 a Identify the needs, background and experiences of the individuals for whom you are providing a home.
HSC350 a, b + c Recognise, respect and support the spiritual well-being of individuals.
HSC3111 a + b Promote equality, diversity rights and responsibilities of individuals.
HSC3116 a, b + c Contribute to promoting a culture that values and respects the diversity of individuals.

Level 4 core units

HSC43 a + b Take responsibility for the continuing professional development of self and others.

Level 4 optional units

HSC414 Assess individual needs and preferences.

Mental Health Standards

D4.1 Identify individuals' needs and circumstances.

F3.1, 3.2, 3.3, 3.4 Prepare and provide agreed individual development activities.

G 8.1, 8.2 Enable people to identify and address their personal spiritual needs.

M3.1, 3.2, 3.3 Contribute to developing and maintaining cultures and strategies in which people are respected and valued as individuals.

Care Homes for Older People: National Minimum Standards

7.1 to 7.6 These standards relate to an individualised plan of care based on a comprehensive assessment to ensure individualised care.

10.3 Service users wear their own clothes at all times.

14.1 to 14.5 These standards relate to allowing clients to exercise choice and control over their lives.

Further reading and references

Chapman, A., Jaques, A. and Marshall, M. (1999) *Dementia Care: 2nd edition. A Handbook for Residential and Day Care.* London: Age Concern.

Cheston, R. and Bender, M. (1999) *Understanding Dementia: The Man with the Worried Eyes.* London: Jessica Kingsley Publishers.

This is a very comprehensive and readable book outlining a very person centred approach to care. It gives a good background introduction to dementia and its effects. See especially Chapter 14, 'Identity work', which describes ways of helping clients to retain a sense of individuality.

Goldsmith, M. (1997) 'Hearing their voice.' In S. Hunter (ed) *Dementia: Challenges and New Directions.* Research Highlights in Social Work 31. London: Jessica Kingsley Publishers.

This looks at the importance of listening to the dementia sufferer and getting their history and story.

Kitwood, T. (1997a) *Dementia Reconsidered: The Person Comes First.* Buckingham: Open University Press.

The whole of this book is excellent but see in particular Chapter 1 'On being a person' and Chapter 3 'How personhood is undermined' – this describes the manner and effects of bad care. Chapter 4, 'Personhood maintained', and Chapter 6, 'Improving care: The next step forward', describes what can be done to enhance personhood and well-being.

Kitwood, T. (1997b) 'Personhood, dementia and dementia care.' In S. Hunter (ed.) *Dementia: Challenges and New Directions.* Research Highlights in Social Work 31. London: Jessica Kingsley Publishers.

This gives a potted history of dementia care and outlines the modern attitude to care.

Pritchard, J. (2003) *A Training Manual for Working with Older People in Residential and Day Care Settings.* London: Jessica Kingsley Publishers.

This is a guide to good practice in elder care with a good section on basic principles of caring, rights and individuality.

Exercise 6.1

YOU!

It is worth just spending some time pondering what it is about yourself that marks you off as an individual. What makes you different from everybody else and stops you from being a clone? What makes you tick? What is really important in your life?

- Just spend a few minutes thinking about these issues and write down your answers.

- Write down ten things which in combination make you a unique individual.

- Then ask to what degree you could answer the same questions for your clients. It is these important aspects of life that we need to know about if we are to be able to treat our clients as individuals.

Exercise 6.2

INDIVIDUALITY

Get together with your colleagues and make a list of all your clients on a flip chart or white board. Next to each name write down the characteristics which set that person apart from the rest. Try to dig out as much of their individuality as possible. When you are happy that you have a good list, discuss it with any relatives or friends of theirs so that they can add their perceptions. They might have noticed something which you did not or might be aware of factors you were not sure of. Having done this, get together again and for each client brain storm ways in which you can actively foster and promote this individuality by the care you give. How can you encourage it and in what ways can you change your care in order to help this?

✓

Exercise 6.3

ROUTINE

With a group of colleagues brain storm ways in which you think life in a residential or nursing home can erode or undermine the individuality of clients. What aspects of life in the home are the key elements of this? List the tasks you perform on a daily basis and look at their impact upon individuality. Write down a job list for your typical day, a sort of detailed job description, and scrutinise this. Look at each of the activities of daily living such as washing, dressing, eating and sleeping in order to assess the opportunity to identify ways in which a bit more individuality can be put back. Go through this list in relation to each client.

Exercise 6.4

VARIETY

- How far does your establishment allow for individual variation?

- Think about whether you ask about the client's normal routines when they are admitted and what effect not being able to stick to these routines will have on the client.

Exercise 6.5

STRENGTHS

List each client in turn and brain storm a list of that client's strengths, skills and positive attributes such as a sense of humour or a liking for sorting, rummaging, singing or gardening. Now for each client think of ways in which you can nurture and use these talents in ways which will give them a sense of being involved and of being successful and useful.

Exercise 6.6

TAKEN FOR GRANTED

Offering choices and delivering individual preferences is a key way of achieving individual care. Can you think of ways in which you make decisions for your clients?

Go through each aspect of the daily routine to check for those things you take for granted. Examples might be choosing what clients wear, what they eat, when to have a cup of tea. The list will probably be a lot longer than you imagined.

Once you have come up with the list, sit down as a group and try and work your way through it, attempting to come up with ways in which you could offer choice.

Exercise 6.7

PROVIDING OPPORTUNITY

Jacki Pritchard (2003) has described a series of everyday events which sometimes are denied to our clients in care. They are things most of us take for granted in our lives, such as having a drink, shopping, keeping a pet, having sex, bathing when we want to or not, going to bed when we want.

- Generate a list with your colleagues of aspects of your life, choices and options which are not available to your clients.

- Discuss how you might be able to offer the same choices and options to clients.

- How does the fact that your clients have dementia affect their enjoyment of these rights and opportunities?

- Should the fact that they have dementia affect this opportunity and if they are denied certain choices, then why do they not have these opportunities?

- Take each one in turn and examine what provision you might make for the client to experience these rights.

Exercise 6.8

WHY?

- It sounds obvious but, with colleagues, just brain storm a list of reasons for spending some time each day with clients on an individual basis.

- List the benefits for the client and the benefits for you.

Exercise 6.9

TALKING POINTS

List two topics each of your clients is interested in, about which you could strike up a conversation. If clients cannot speak, identify two ways of sharing time on an individual basis that they would enjoy. This might be looking at pictures or simply holding hands: the list of possibilities is endless. You will need to know your clients quite well to come up with a list that works here.

Exercise 6.10
OBSERVATIONS AND ASSUMPTIONS

To get a feel for what a history can do, try this observations and assumptions exercise.

- Get together with one of your work colleagues whom you do not know very well.

- Have a chat about work-related issues such as any current problems or issues around how to improve the quality of care.

- Do not talk about each other or personal issues. Chat for about ten minutes.

- After chatting sit back to back and try to answer the following questions about them:

  - Are they wearing any jewellery?
  - Describe their hairstyle and colour.
  - Describe their eyes.
  - How old are they?
  - What height and weight are they?
  - What are they wearing?
  - What do you imagine their favourite food to be?
  - If they ordered a drink in a bar what would it be?
  - What magazines do they read?
  - What newspaper do they take?
  - What are their politics?
  - Are they religious?
  - What hobbies do they have?
  - What do they do in their spare time?
  - What is their idea of a good night out?
  - What do they watch on TV?
  - Are they married?
  - Do they have children?
  - Do they keep pets?
  - What do you imagine makes them tick?

- Write down the answers on a piece of paper and then feed back to each other what you have written.

- Check out each other's assumptions and how accurate or not they are.

You might be surprised at what you found out here!

INDIVIDUAL CLIENT PROFILE

Personal details

Full name and title

What do they like to be called?

Date and place of birth

Most recent home address

Next of kin

Contact details of significant others; frequency of contact

Partner

Children (with date of birth)

Siblings

Friends

Other

Notable dates

Family birthdays, anniversaries, major life landmarks, etc.

Home life

Where did they live? History since school, married/courting, parenting, pets, housework, budgeting, cooking, shopping, DIY, etc.

Personal care

Hygiene needs and preferences

Bath or shower routines

Dental care

Use of toiletries, favourites

Childhood

Where were they brought up? What was it like?

Education

School: did they like it or not? What was it like? School friends? Were they 'good'?
Games? Favourite subjects?

College and university

Other

Sex and affection
How were these needs fulfilled?

Culture/Religion
Customs

Beliefs

Privacy, hygiene, food

Gender issues

Are they actively religious: do they keep a faith and how do they practise it?

Need for prayer or services

When are key religious dates/festivals and how do they celebrate them?

Politics
Importance to them

Practices and need to participate

Work

What jobs did they have from school onwards, what was last career, did they love it or loathe it?

Any special skills and achievements?

Values and beliefs

What are these and how did they adhere to these in practice?

Interest in current affairs and news

Newspaper read

Interests and hobbies

Which sports did they enjoy and how did they participate? Favourite teams?

Indoor pursuits: TV, radio, games, puzzles, bingo, craftwork, reading, etc.

Outdoor pursuits: Walking, gardening, birdwatching, riding, driving, etc.

Visiting friends/Entertaining

Arts: cinema, theatre, other

Travel: holiday preferences and outings; where have they been?

Wartime or military experience

What, when and significance

Heroes

Anyone they particularly admired from childhood onwards

Coping

How did they cope in a crisis? What did they do when they needed comforting?

Routines adhered to

Mealtimes

Morning and bedtimes, evenings

Others

General likes and dislikes

Food and drink, breakfast, dinner, tea and supper; snacks; alcohol

Clothing: How do they like to dress? What particular style? Favourite clothes, use of jewellery and other adornments, make-up, hairstyle, shoes

Music and TV, favourite singers, composers, favourite TV shows, favourite films

Company and activity

Others

Favourite possessions

Keepsakes, pictures, photos, ornaments and souvenirs, music, books, jewellery

✓

Exercise 6.12

SELF-ASSESSMENT

In order for you to get an idea of the kind of information required and see the need for detail, photocopy the form and do a profile of yourself. Have in mind what it is you would want carers to know about you.

Having done this, read it through and give it to a friend to look at to see if there is anything they think is important about you that you have left out. Ask them if there is anything about you that they did not know.

Exercise 6.13

AMBITIONS

- What are your client's ambitions?

- Did you think they had any?

- Clients with dementia can still have goals that they want to achieve. Find out what these are and help them to work towards achieving them.

Exercise 6.14

WHO AM I?

This is an exercise in how well you know any individual client. First, though, you need to do it for yourself.

- Write a list of the 20 most important aspects of your life. For example:

    ◦ I am married to…
    ◦ I am the father of…
    ◦ I like to…
    ◦ I am a supporter of…
    ◦ I own…
    ◦ I work as…
    ◦ Include all those people and things that are important to you and make you happy, such as hobbies and passions.

- Now write the list for any of your clients and see if any of these aspects need to be better incorporated or catered for in your care in order to account for the client's individuality.

Chapter 7

Activity

Key messages

- The most important activities are those that include one in ordinary life, such as making the bed, washing the car, shopping and doing the laundry or washing the dishes.
- Art and craft, outings and other activities will significantly boost clients' stimulation and interaction and are easy to organise and do.
- Care workers need to act as advocates for clients to ensure that management support staff in doing such activity.

The importance of stimulating and meaningful activity cannot be understated. The main emphasis should be upon inclusion and fun but other major benefits are the relief of boredom and maintenance of self-esteem, plus the preservation of physical, cognitive and social skills. Where activity levels are high you are also likely to see a marked reduction in restlessness and agitation. Confusion on the part of a client need not be a barrier to participation: many activities can be adapted to be failure free if someone who suffers from severe confusion is involved. Inclusion in even the simplest tasks will give clients a meaningful role and even something as mundane as drying cutlery with a tea towel can be a pleasurable experience for them in the company of a skilled care worker.

Such an interaction will give clients a sense of companionship. It will also be an opportunity to practise social and communication skills. There will be valuable physical exercise involved but, most important, the client will be made to feel useful and wanted. A care worker with imagination can even reverse the caring role with the client doing things for them instead of the usual scenario of the client having things done to and for them.

Activity is not just about art and crafts and trips out in the minibus. By far the most important aspect is inclusion in 'everyday' or 'normal' life. Helping with the washing up, putting clothes in the washing machine, shopping, washing the car, vacuuming – these are all examples of the many activities in which clients can be included. Carers must be creative and identify opportunities for including clients. Most care homes, for example, have a newspaper delivered, but this could so easily be changed to a client taking a daily stroll with a care worker to the newsagent to buy it. This gives the client a useful role, some exercise and fresh air. The important thing is that they are still needed, still a part of normal life.

Alongside such 'normal' activity remains the need to organise activity sessions which should break up the day. Skilled carers can encourage participation from clients who would otherwise receive little stimulation. The nightmare scenario is one of people sitting around the outside of the room, not interacting at all during a day punctuated only by mealtimes or the need for the toilet. Imagine the boredom of such a scenario repeated day after day.

Making a difference

A key to success in activity planning is in knowing your clients. You can then tailor the activity to suit their abilities and interests. You might have to try several different activities before you find those which are successful. However, it is worth persevering because it will allow you to develop a routine of those activities which work well. Life can be very boring for residents, and often the most important and stimulating activities are mealtimes. What you must ask yourself is the question 'How can I make today more interesting and special? How can I make it different from yesterday?' (see Exercises 7.1 and 7.2, p.68).

Important considerations
Appropriateness

You must ensure that the activity matches the ability of the person so that they can join in. Don't set severely confused clients up for failure by giving them activities which are way beyond their capabilities. On the other hand don't give simplistic tasks, well below the ability of the person, because this will be demeaning and insulting. It is also important that the activities are age appropriate and not childish. Many children's activities can be adapted, though, and used in a way which is not demeaning.

Fun

Make it fun! Confusion is no barrier to laughter. In fact if you can make one hour a day funny, or at least light-hearted, then you will have achieved much towards making your clients' lives happier.

Groups

Many activities are important for their social nature but if you want to begin some group work remember to keep groups small so that you can give attention to and include all participants. Working in groups can help to foster a sense of togetherness and help group members to get to know each other better. Developing such a sense of community can enhance the experience of institutional living. Remember that there are those who will not be used to group activity and you will need to find out what works for your clients. Eventually though you will build up a range of activities that most will enjoy and that can be repeated on a regular basis.

Pace

Take your time; don't rush. This is a key factor in the success of any activity. You must go at the clients' speed and for this reason it's best not to have too wide an ability range within the group. Mixing people with early dementia and people with late stage dementia will mean that your activity is easy for some, difficult for some and at the right level for just a few. It is also worth remembering that in dementia attention span can be short, so keep activities brief in order that they remain enjoyable.

Emphasis

Remember, the end result is not as important as the participation and fun involved. Do not get too concerned about the finished product of an art or craft session: what really matters is that people were involved and some sort of social interaction was had. Clients need to feel they have been part of something rather than just doing something!

Simplicity, familiarity and repetition

Keep things simple by breaking them down into small steps. Most activities are achievable in this way. It is also important to use activities based upon previous lifestyles and hobbies and skills. Find out what people used to like doing and see if these skills can be rekindled. There may be an ability to play a musical instrument or football, or an enthusiasm for fashion, which is being overlooked. With advanced dementia, it is often useful to use activities which involve repetition such as sorting and arranging things. Simply rummaging together through a box of odds and ends can be pleasurable when it is used to give praise and as a communication opportunity. Such activities can all give a sense of doing something useful.

Praise

Give praise frequently for even the smallest effort made by a client as it is a huge stimulus and boost to self-esteem. Use verbal and non-verbal methods, smiles, hugs, claps, etc. Remember that your enthusiasm is a prime motivator and it will be crucial in motivating others, both clients and fellow staff.

Relevant

Try to use activities based on the person's previous interests; get to know who loved cooking, gardening, bingo, crafts, housework etc. The cardinal rules apply again – get to know your clients' histories.

Inclusion

It is very important to emphasise this point. Even the most severely confused client can be included in activities in some way by skilled carers. Often all it takes is keeping things simple and allowing clients time to do them. For example, if you are tidying up someone's room, take that person with you, talk to them, get them to hold something or do some dusting or fold some clothes. This simple scenario will give the person interaction, recognition, a role, companionship. Give praise for even the smallest of achievements, even if it's just being there for a few minutes with you. The only limit to inclusion is your imagination and enthusiasm. Focus on the ordinary things people do in everyday life, such as washing up or cleaning, and use these as activities to keep people involved.

Suggestions for successful activity

Music

Music is very powerful; it seems to linger in the memory and trigger a whole host of associations from the past. Often people who are reluctant to join in other activities will derive much pleasure from singing along to, or simply listening to, familiar and favourite tunes in the company of others. Easy to organise, sing-along sessions are frequently the most successful of activities. Logistically they are good because they can be enjoyed from the comfort of the armchair. The carer's participation and enthusiasm during the session will be of enormous encouragement to the clients here. You will soon find your group's favourite songs and you can discuss the memories these trigger. You can also introduce the idea of dancing. These sessions are often so much fun that they can be repeated frequently. Every so often it will be possible to organise special tea dances or themed sing-along sessions.

Exercise

This is one of the easiest activities to arrange. Simply going out for a walk with a client will provide a brief interlude of exercise, stimulation and social contact. In a small group a simple gentle exercise session can form an enjoyable part of a daily routine which is easy to organise. Such a group also encourages social interaction. You might be able to ask your local physiotherapist to devise a routine for your clients. With luck they may be able to come along once in a while to conduct their own sessions. Other good ideas are throwing a soft ball around to each other, aiming bean bags at a target in the middle of the room and games such as skittles. All of these can be done while sitting in an armchair and all can be adapted so that everyone can join in.

Food

People can be included here in many ways such as food preparation, cooking, baking, laying the tables and other kitchen and dining-room activities. Try to include clients in as many aspects as possible. Simple recipes for biscuits and cakes can be followed and if they are broken down into small steps there is no reason why anyone should be excluded. You can work with individuals or in groups, having a baking group for example. If any birthdays or special events are coming up, use this as a focus for the group, or just use the results of your baking as an excuse for a party. It doesn't matter if you end up doing much of it yourself: you will have included people and made something different happen.

Art and craft

Almost anything in this category can be adapted and simplified, but avoid anything too complicated. It is important to keep things at an adult level: you can use children's art and craft equipment and kits but do it in an adult way. Again the end product is not so important; it's the inclusion and the social aspects that come first. Some good ideas that are failure-free are creating leaf and dried-flower pictures, making greeting cards, plaster moulding, painting and colouring. The range of possibilities is enormous and these activities can be done in groups or in one-to-one sessions. A simple colouring session using photocopied pictures can be very successful and inclusive.

Collage

One of the best art activities is the collage: there is little preparation, it's easy and the results look good. It is also a good activity because you can include almost anybody. Simply looking through a variety of magazines together and discussing the pictures people like is the first part of the process. Then with some cutting and pasting decide where to place them and build up your picture, sticking the magazine pictures onto a large coloured sheet. Try making collages with specific themes such as animals, places, people, gardens and seasons. This activity will also allow you to reminisce while you make the collage. There can be a lot of social interaction in making a collage and the end result can be proudly displayed and changed on a regular basis.

Scrapbook

Working with individuals you can build up a scrapbook which will provide a useful and personal reminiscence resource. These should be a sort of 'This is Your Life', full of mementos, family photos etc., to be shared and read together on a regular basis. You can also make themed scrapbooks for use as reminiscence tools. Themes could be animals, plants, places, people etc. Make them in group sessions, sharing the task and generating interaction. These are useful resources for just sitting with individuals and looking at the pictures together when you have just a few minutes to spare.

Gardens

Merely spending time looking at the garden together will give companionship, exercise and fresh air. Many aspects of tending the garden, such as weeding, can be shared and small projects such as window boxes can be undertaken together. Other jobs that can be shared out are watering plants and tending to the bird table.

Solo and one-to-one

It is important not to relegate activity to weekly group sessions. You should also allow time for regular one-to-one sessions with individual clients. This is especially true with regard to reminiscence and helping with ordinary household chores.

Others

There are many good activity books (Briscoe 1991; Dowling 1995; Perrin and May 1999; Sherman 1991; Walsh 1993) that contain many other activities you can try out. Other tried-and-tested activities are outings, bingo, building up a photograph album, looking at magazines together, shopping, going for a drive, guessing games such as hiding an object in a pillow case and then getting people to try and guess what it is. Many people have had hobbies and were good at certain things such as woodwork and knitting; get to know which of your clients fall into these categories and provide them with the opportunity to continue these skills. Finally, there will be times when you need to do something quick – it's a good idea to have a 'memory box' full of old objects, photos, postcards and in fact anything that can be discussed and passed around. Keep adding to it and you will have a useful short-notice activity. Experiment!

Think

Thinking might be the most important thing you ever do in terms of improving the quality of life of clients in your care. Ask yourself for each client: 'How can I include them more in the daily routine? How can I include them more in taking care of their own needs? What activities can I do with them?' Without activity life is not enjoyable. Without enjoyment life is meaningless. Imagine doing nothing for a day, then all week, then imagine if the previous week had been the same. You would quickly become depressed and deskilled. Activity and interaction make us tick.

Sensory therapy

Activity that focuses on sensory stimulation can be very useful in advanced dementia. As cognitive abilities decline the ability to communicate via the senses becomes more important. We can effectively use the senses to give people a feeling of reassurance by hugging them and smiling when they can no longer understand our words of reassurance. We know that the senses remain largely intact in dementia and so we can use this as a focus for activities. Music, massage, aromas, touch, colours, pictures etc. can all be used creatively and therapeutically to provide a pleasurable experience and a communication opportunity. A major benefit of such sessions is likely to be a sense of relaxation and a reduction in anxiety. Multi-sensory Snoezelen rooms use bubble machines, music, projections, fibre optics, tactile materials etc. The object here is to share pleasant experiences with clients and to communicate that shared pleasure. There are many other opportunities to use the senses which are often overlooked. Having a box of materials which are soft and comforting to feel can provide an opportunity for sharing as can a simple massage and aromatherapy.

Health and Social Care National Occupational Standards

This chapter relates to many of the induction and foundation standards but in particular to the following level standards:

Level 2 core units

HSC23 b Use new and improved skills and knowledge in your work.

Level 2 optional units

HSC210 a, b + c Support individuals to access and participate in recreational activities.
HSC211 a, b + c Support individuals to take part in developmental activities.
HSC228 b Contribute to the implementation of group care programmes and activities.

Level 3 optional units

HSC331 a, b + c Support individuals to develop and maintain social networks and relationships.
HSC393 a, b + c Prepare, implement and evaluate therapeutic group activities.

Level 4 optional units

HSC420 a + b Promote leisure opportunities and activities for individuals.

Mental Health Standards

F1.1, 1.2, 1.3 Prepare, implement and evaluate agreed therapeutic group activities.

F3.1, 3.2, 3.3, 3.4 Prepare and provide agreed individual development activities.

G9.1, 9.2 Enable people to choose and participate in activities which are meaningful to them.

H4.1, 4.2 Support people in relation to personal and social interactions and environmental factors.

Care Homes for Older People: National Minimum Standards

12.1, 12.2, 12.3 and 12.4 These standards relate to the provision of a choice of social and leisure activity which is flexible and varied to suit the service user's expectations, preferences and capacities. Clients' interests should be recorded and opportunities to meet these needs should be available within and outside the home environment. The standard states that particular consideration should be given to clients with dementia.

Further reading and references

Briscoe, T. (1991) *Develop an Activities Programme*. Bicester: Winslow Press.

Dowling, J.R. (1995) *Keeping Busy: A Handbook of Activities for Persons with Dementia*. Baltimore: John Hopkins University Press.

Johnson, A. (1998) 'All play and no work? Take a fresh look at activities.' *Journal of Dementia Care*. Nov/Dec, 25–7.

Perrin, T. and May, H. (1999) *Well-being in Dementia: An Occupational Approach for Therapists and Carers*. London: Churchill Livingstone.

Sherman, M. (1991) *The Reminiscence Quiz Book*. Bicester: Winslow Press.

Walsh, D. (1993) *Groupwork Activities: The Manual for Those Working with the Elderly*. Bicester: Winslow Press.

This is useful as a source of many group and individual activities. It is a vast collection of activities. They vary from those with an essentially therapeutic end to those that are easy to organise and largely social in nature. There is an emphasis upon activities that are suitable for older adults suffering with mental health problems and special emphasis is given to activities that can be successfully carried out with people suffering dementia.

Exercise 7.1

GENERATING IDEAS

Arrange a meeting with colleagues to think about the activities you provide or do not. What is it that gets in the way of providing stimulating activity? The lack of mental stimulation and endurance of long periods of inactivity is one of the commonest and most overlooked forms of *abuse* in current residential and nursing home practice. The argument that dementia makes it difficult cannot be used as an excuse here. It *is* possible to engage with and stimulate clients even in the advanced stages of dementia. Under-stimulation and inactivity should not be tolerated in any setting. So discuss in the group what gets in the way of doing more activities and what you might do to improve the situation.

Taking each of the major categories of activity, such as music, art and craft, food, exercise, outdoor activity, reminiscence and games, consider how you might introduce them into your daily schedule. Try looking at your clients one by one and come up with ideas for activities that they might enjoy individually, as activity does not have to be done in groups.

Debate these ideas and then try to put them together into some sort of workable plan. This is important as if you do not identify when the activity should occur and who should do it then invariably it will not happen. Usually both clients and carers benefit as life becomes more interesting for both. After a while a pattern of successful sessions will emerge which can be built upon.

Exercise 7.2

EVERYDAY LIFE

- Write a list of everything each client does such as get up, get dressed, have a wash, eat breakfast, etc. Do this for their whole day.

- Next write a list of everything you do throughout an average shift.

- Now, for each list, think about ways in which you could offer choices or maximise inclusion and encourage the client to do more for themselves.

Chapter 8

Therapeutic Relationships, Reality Orientation, Validation and Resolution Approaches

Key messages

- It is not what you do but how you do it that is most important.
- Building up a relationship with clients is crucial and this means finding out about their past and just 'being with' them, spending time with them.

The importance of a good therapeutic relationship

The importance of a good therapeutic relationship can never be understated in mental health nursing. It is the most important aspect of care. If you fail to build up a therapeutic relationship with a client then whatever else you try to do has a much diminished chance of success. Argyle (1967) suggests that it matters little what theoretical approach you adopt or which therapy you use; what is effective in bringing about change in people's lives is whether or not you can build up a good relationship with the client. If you do build a good rapport with a client then the chances are that other things you try to do will be more effective. The client will be more likely to trust you and work with you. Problems can be more easily resolved too. This is also the case when working with people with dementia. Even in the face of severe cognitive impairment, the better you are at developing a good rapport the better will be the outcome for all. The difference is that in dementia you might have to build that rapport afresh each time you go on duty and each time you interact with the sufferer. Nonetheless, doing this will pay dividends and a carer who puts time and effort into relating, before doing, will make their clients' lives much happier.

Carl Rogers, the founding father of humanistic, person centred counselling, also felt that the relationship between the therapist and the client was essential. Rogers (1951) described certain core conditions which he saw as being essential in a therapeutic relationship:

1. The therapist has *unconditional positive regard* for the client. This means that you respect and accept the client, warts and all. You do not make judgements about them, but value them. This is also sometimes called 'warmth', which is a good way of describing it.

2. The therapist has an *empathic* understanding of the client's world and experience. This is much deeper than sympathy: it is an attempt to try and see the world as the client sees it, to understand what they are actually experiencing.

3. The therapist must be *genuine* and honest, open and frank. You should be yourself, not some starchy professional. Show your human side. Give reasons for disagreeing where you do not see eye to eye. Explain all you do.

4. The therapist can *communicate* these qualities to the client.

These skills are essential to good care and forming a relationship with clients. The use of counselling skills such as reflection form a key element when communicating with confused clients. 'Reflection' is merely, stating back to the client in your own words (or even using the same words) what they have said to you. This gives the client with dementia the opportunity to check that you have understood. In the latter stages of dementia, just being warm and present can sometimes be enough.

Listening

Other key counselling skills are crucial. Listening skills are perhaps the most vital. Being with and listening to sufferers gives them the feeling that they are still important and valued. It allows them a base from which to begin to explore just what it is that is happening to them. Being listened to will lessen their isolation and give them a sense of relief at being recognised as being in trauma; it makes the nightmare more tolerable. The 'active' listener should be listening for the feelings being expressed as well as the verbal message. Good listening also means paying attention to non-verbal aspects, such as facial expression and posture, and comfort behaviours, such as rocking or shaking a foot or arm. These convey the inner state of the person and raw emotions such as anger, happiness and sadness.

Thus, simple ways to form a therapeutic relationship with confused clients would be to always greet them and use their names. Use touch as appropriate since this can convey your sincerity and it implies friendliness and warmth. Be aware of the communication guidelines as set out in Chapter 5 and remember to go at their pace.

Therapies

Within the context of a good therapeutic relationship and using counselling skills, it is important to look at the concepts of Reality Orientation, Validation Therapy and Resolution Therapy and how they fit in with each other. In general, in the early stages of dementia, when short-term memory is still useable, it is appropriate to use Reality Orientation in order to try and retain the client's independence. However, as the illness progresses and short-term memory fades, there comes a time when reorientation becomes pointless. It then becomes more useful to use validation and resolution approaches to communication (see Figure 8.1).

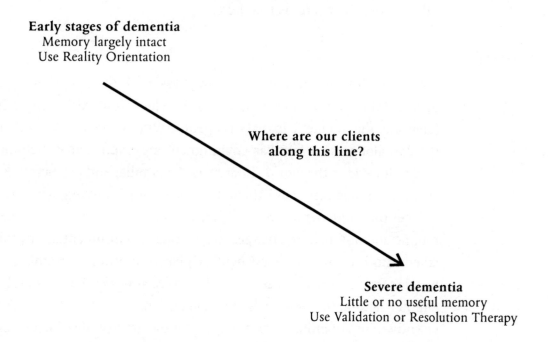

Early stages of dementia
Memory largely intact
Use Reality Orientation

Where are our clients along this line?

Severe dementia
Little or no useful memory
Use Validation or Resolution Therapy

Figure 8.1 Progression of an Alzheimer's type dementia

Figure 8.1 represents the progress of an Alzheimer's type dementia. The important thing for us, as carers, is to get to know our clients so that we can judge where they are on this line.

Reality Orientation

The aim of Reality Orientation (RO) is to help clients to maintain a grasp on reality and thus remain independent and able to perform activities of daily living. It is important that clients retain their grasp on reality with respect to time, place, person and the who, what, where, when and how of life. To do this there are several different forms which RO can take.

24-HOUR REALITY ORIENTATION

This is a sort of running commentary on the day and what is happening, constant re-affirmation and reinforcement. It is the continual provision of verbal clues and cues which allows the sufferer to remain aware of what it is they need to do. Typically, information given by the carer might take the form of a continuous dialogue while, for example, helping someone in the morning. 'Here John, this is your sock, it goes on your foot, here, like this.' The carer in this scenario has mimed the action to remind John who was struggling to remember, but who subsequently gets it right and so puts on his other sock unaided. This would continue throughout the day with carers constantly providing John with the necessary clues and information to be as independent as possible. The maxim 'silent care is bad care' is true here.

ROUTINE

We are all glued to routines! Wake up, dress, walk the dog, shave, put the kettle on, etc. Taking away our familiar cues and clues would disorient us in much the same way that memory loss affects people with dementia. A familiar routine to the day alongside a familiar environment are important in helping clients to remain located in the world. Take away the familiar and problems arise. Altering clients' routines can cause them anxiety in not knowing what to do next; it reduces their independence too. Thus an important part of RO is maintaining a routine and not making changes to a familiar environment. Many clients, when taken into hospital for assessment or placed in a home to give carers respite, become much more confused than they were at home. This is simply the loss of familiar landmarks (where is the toilet?), change to routine and fear of the unknown. In unfamiliar surroundings people get lost, disoriented, agitated and upset.

LABELLING

By labelling doors, rooms and drawers etc. with large signs or pictures in order to remind the client of what lies within, you help to maintain their independence. Use signs first, then pictures when the client no longer recognises words – it appears that the ability to understand pictures is retained longer than the ability to read words.

A classic example of the benefits of labelling relates to incontinence. Carers had noticed that Joshua had had several accidents and his urinary incontinence was becoming almost regular. He became doubly incontinent. Staff noticed an increase in agitation which they eventually linked to his need to go to the toilet. Joshua's incontinence was medically investigated but no cause could be found. The simple fact was that he had forgotten where the toilet was. Thus a large sign, 'TOILET', was stuck to the toilet door and Joshua instantly became continent again.

Several months later the pattern recurred with Joshua becoming incontinent again. This time he could no longer make sense of the words on the door and the sign was meaningless to him, so he quickly forgot where the toilet was. Replacing the sign with a picture of a toilet instantly restored his continence and independence.

Labelling clothes drawers, cutlery cupboards etc. all helps the sufferer to locate things and so remain independent rather then having to rely on others. Pictures of milk on the fridge door, socks and pants on the relevant drawers in the bedroom – these are very simple but very effective methods of prolonging someone's independence. Large clocks and calendars are another example of labelling.

REALITY ORIENTATION BOARDS

RO boards are to be found in many wards, day centres and nursing homes. Essentially they are white boards with details of place, date, weather, staff, menus and activities etc. They are important in providing sufferers with a point of reference and a reminder of basic information: they help them to get their bearings.

COLOUR CODING

This is sometimes seen in hospitals with coloured lines along the walls: 'Follow the green line to the x-ray department'. More commonly in residential and nursing homes specific doors are coloured, thus all the toilet doors might be red and all the bedrooms green.

REALITY ORIENTATION GROUPS

Formal RO sessions can be run in groups with a varied focus. They can be a mixture of both RO and reminiscence. The group may, for example, discuss the cold weather and winter after some name and place reminders, and then go on to reminisce about winter. It is vitally important to take into account the level of cognitive impairment within the group. It will be fine to discuss the 'winter' in the group with clients in the early stages of dementia, but if clients are in the latter stages then the information will be too difficult and not mean anything to them and you will only succeed in making them feel a sense of failure for not understanding. Those above the level of the group will be insulted and patronised. There is also the possibility that they may be frightened: sufferers in more advanced stages may provide them with an insight into what might lie ahead for themselves. You must ensure that group members are all at a similar level. Generally RO groups should have an emphasis on fun and be fairly short. They should also be small and frequent. A good knowledge of your group members' pasts will help to make the group more relevant and personal.

PERSONAL HISTORY BOARDS AND SCRAPBOOKS

History boards and scrapbooks are a great idea. The idea behind both records is to maintain the client's grasp on their own identity. History boards are pin boards placed by bedsides or in prominent places in clients' rooms. A blend of RO and reminiscence, they contain the client's name, photographs of the client and family members, mementos of life, work and hobbies, pictures of pets and favourite things. The board might also have club cards and travel passes and photos of other important aspects of the client's life, such as pets and hobbies, pinned to it. It is a reference to themselves and can form a regular source of conversation with carers and a reminder to clients. Personal scrapbooks take this idea further. Basically you collate a scrapbook of the person's life to use in one-to-one sessions focusing on their past and current identity. See Chapters 6 and 9 on client history and reminiscence for further details.

Validation Therapy

Validation Therapy is complimentary to RO, not a replacement for it. The two therapies should be used at different stages of the illness. In the latter stages of dementia, when the sufferer is experiencing further cognitive decline, short-term memory will reach the point where it is virtually non-existent. At this stage the information and clues provided by RO will not be recognised or retained long enough to be useful. It becomes meaningless to talk about the date and to try and reinforce our reality with respect to place, time and other everyday details. It is, however, worth maintaining a focus on the person with respect to who they are. The person may not be able to remember or respond but doing this will help carers to retain a sense of the individual rather than beginning to see only the dementia. In a sense we remember who the sufferers are *for* them, because they can no longer do it. Thus I would want you to remember that I am a dad who loved walking and wildlife, long after I have lost interest. You need to retain my sense of me for me!

When the client has little short-term memory left, their long-term memory is brought to the fore and often they seem to be living in the past. Without the benefit of short-term memory, this past becomes where they are. The client has only ideas, connections, thoughts and images from the past in their minds and so it is the reality for them. It is real and current to them. Typically the sufferer thinks that they are 30 years old as opposed to being 80-something years. They may feel that they have just been demobbed from the armed forces or have just gone to the shops to get a loaf of bread for 'Mum'. Just think about this for a minute. If you believed that to be the case, what would you make of what was going on around you in a modern twenty-first century nursing home? It is likely that you would be frightened, and it is also likely that you might feel that you were being imprisoned or had been abducted. Compounding this would be the experience of being forcibly held against your will. It is easy to see why some clients become very scared and agitated.

It would be pointless to try RO with clients at this stage. 'Hello John, my name's Danny, I am a nurse; this is Green Gables, a nursing home, this is where you live now.' The simple fact is that the client is locked into his/her reality and it is pointless to try and enforce ours. Doing so can have disturbing implications. An 83-year-old lady, Mary, feels that she needs to get home. In her reality, she is 16 and has gone out on an errand and is late back. She tells you that her mum will 'kill her' if she is any later. According to Mary, she *is* 16, so to use RO and tell her that she is 83 would be tantamount to telling her that her mother is dead. You run the risk of putting Mary through serial grief reactions by reinforcing your reality. Mary might not retain the information long, but you are telling her, for the first time, that her mother is dead every time you use RO.

At these later stages of dementia a Validation Therapy approach is more appropriate. This essentially suggests that you should disregard the obvious unreality to you and try and understand the reality from the client's point of view. You should validate their experience of reality. Thus, in the case of Mary, you should accept her fears and try and communicate with her about what it feels like to be 16 and late home. Get her to talk about her mum and console her about her fears. In this way you are acknowledging her reality rather than dismissing it. That reality is all our clients have, and if we do not validate it, if we dismiss it, this is tantamount to telling them that they do not exist, they are not important. In effect you destroy their world. The carer's ability to enter the world of the client at this stage is crucial to good care. The carer must acknowledge the content of what is said and engage with the client according to that reality, but, more important, the carer must validate the feelings being expressed by the client.

Another fact of dementia is that, while many cognitive functions decline, the ability to feel and express feelings and emotions remains intact. The one thing you can know for certain is that the only method of communication that is still open to access is via feelings. *Feelings are paramount.* Clients with dementia still experience feelings and emotions as we all do and they still express them in the same way. Thus a client who cries is sad, a client who laughs is happy. So even if we cannot understand clients' words or work out what it is they are saying, we can still be certain of their emotional states and validate them by laughing with them or putting our arms around them and hugging them in their sadness.

The 'inventor' of Validation Therapy, Naomi Feil, suggests that by living in the past, clients are somehow trying to resolve 'unfinished emotional conflicts'. This, however, seems unlikely, as in the latter stages of a dementia clients simply do not have the cognitive ability to organise such a review of past relationships. It has also been suggested that clients revert to past times as a way of escaping a present they can make no sense of. But it is not a conscious decision to revert to past times. It is simply that the long-term memory has become the only point of reference now that short-term memory no longer exists. In effect the present does not exist. However, the basic message of validation – that we should validate the client's reality and support the feelings they express – represents a valuable approach for carers when clients are beyond the reach of Reality Orientation.

Resolution Therapy

Counselling skills such as active listening are essential to Resolution Therapy, as described by Goudie and Stokes (1990). Resolution Therapy uses reflective listening to help sufferers to express their feelings; it does this by urging carers to try to recognise and empathise with the feelings being expressed in any verbal message. Doing this will help clients to feel that their feelings are recognised and acknowledged, as using Validation Therapy did. The difference is that Resolution Therapy also suggests that within any confused communication there is always a hidden message or a concealed meaning. Any utterance, no matter how bizarre to us, will have real meaning for the client and it is up to us to try and guess it: we only have to listen carefully to work out what it is. Thus we must validate the feelings being expressed and also try to guess the hidden meanings behind what is said no matter how nonsensical to us. The goal in Resolution Therapy is to achieve a sense of well-being and recognise that 'feelings are paramount'.

This approach has at its heart a desire to preserve the dignity of the individual by accepting the reality of the client and attempting to validate it. Such validation and its acknowledgement of the client's feeling must be comforting for clients when so much else around them makes little or no sense. The skills involved in trying to find hidden meanings will also underpin such support and benefit the client. The Resolution Therapy approach recognises the value of basic counselling skills, so the carer will display warmth and acceptance. Carers should also explore the client's feelings and reflect them back to the client, while striving to find ways to resolve such feelings. The resolution is that the client's feelings are recognised, validated and acted upon in a way that brings about a contented or happy conclusion. It is not just about trying to cheer someone up, it is about recognising those feelings and feeding back that we understand how the client feels (empathy). In doing so we validate their feelings, we take them seriously and acknowledge that their feelings are real. If we ignore such feelings we are more or less telling them they are not real persons, they do not matter.

Be intensely aware of body language such as facial expression and posture: they reveal feelings. Like most people, I find it very hard to lie non-verbally, thus non-verbal behaviour is often a window to the soul.

Collusion

If a client says she must go home because her 'mum' is waiting and we say, 'OK I will just finish this and then I will go and get the key', we are colluding with them. A little white lie can be the best method of avoiding painful realisations and awkward situations. However, it is a second-best resort. We should always strive to tell the truth to clients, but would obviously not want to do this if we knew it would cause them much distress. We need to ensure, though, that our collusion does not avoid engaging with the clients' underlying feelings and emotions as in the validation approach. Many nurses and carers do this because it is the easy way out. It is hard to deal with someone's distress at missing their mother, far easier to suggest that it will all soon be all right. Kitwood (Kitwood and Bredin 1991) argues strongly for truth-telling because anything else is building a relationship founded on deception. Most people lie to people they do not respect and who they think are worthless. Often collusion responses are a legacy of a lack of time or an unwillingness to engage with painful emotions. We need to work with clients' feelings and validate them rather than disregard them with a glib lie in the hope that they will forget. By using a lie we are in effect denying them their personhood. We are saying that they do not matter. These are the principles and there will be times when the principles do not match up to the reality of life and work, but if the preservation of dignity and personhood are your guide then your response will always be to validate rather than collude.

An example of collusion would be to say to a distressed resident who was anxious about getting the cows into the barn for the night, 'It's OK, I've seen to it'. An example of validation would be to acknowledge that you recognise the distress and show the client your concern and understanding verbally and non-verbally. You could then validate his reality by trying to get him to talk about how hard life as a farmer can be. If the distress persists then you might have to collude in the end, rather than deny him his reality. It is the collusion without an attempt to validate feelings and the client's reality which is bad practice.

Physical contact

The way you feel is often directly proportional to the amount of positive feedback you get in the way of hugs and kisses. The opportunity for physical contact of a reassuring and loving nature can be limited upon entering an institution. But part of resolution and validation techniques demands a degree of willingness literally to embrace our clients. The emphasis is on recognising feelings and we will invariably unearth many instances of sadness and despair in our clients because dementia is a cruel illness.

We need therefore to be generous with our physical reassurance and validation. A hug can convey what words can't even begin to. And as our clients can't often understand our words, the physical expression of our understanding of their emotional state is crucial. Be mindful of taboos and that some people are not 'tactile' but, essentially, no one can go through life without getting a cuddle every now and again.

Leonard Babins

The expert Leonard Babins (1986) summed up the plight of the sufferer with the insight that sufferers will cope in any way they can with the effects of dementia. Some will withdraw and retreat into their own 'inner cosmos'. Some, he suggests, will constantly doze off in order to avoid the pain of a reality they can no longer grasp. Others will resist or fight their increasing helplessness and display the aggression that is born of frustration. They will yell and scream and be tranquillised or restrained. All options are coping methods and all can be helped by adopting the right approach – be it RO, Validation Therapy or Resolution Therapy. Much of the range of what are often called 'problem behaviours' are attempts to make sense of the world, attempts to communicate with it or just simply and justifiably to rage against it.

Think about the clients you have and whether any of the behaviours they display which are hard to deal with could be born out of the frustration and fear of suffering a dementia.

Health and Social Care National Occupational Standards

This chapter relates to many of the induction and foundation standards but in particular to the following level standards:

Level 2 core units

HSC21 a, b + c Communicate with and complete records for individuals.

Level 2 optional units

HSC26 a, b + c Support individuals to access and use information.
HSC27 a, b + c Support individuals in their daily living.
HSC210 a, b + c Support individuals to access and participate in recreational activities.
HSC212 a, b + c Support individuals during therapy sessions.
HSC233 a, b + c Relate to and interact with individuals.

Level 3 core units

HSC31 a, b + c Promote effective communication for and about individuals.

Level 3 optional units

HSC332 a, b + c Support the social, emotional and identity needs of individuals.

HSC369 a, b + c Support individuals with specific communication needs.

HSC373 a, b + c Plan and implement programmes to enable individuals to find their way around familiar environments.

HSC393 a, b + c Prepare, implement and evaluate agreed therapeutic group activities.

HSC3111 a, b + c Promote the equality, diversity, rights and responsibilities of individuals.

HSC3116 a, b + c Contribute to promoting a culture that values and respects the diversity of individuals.

Level 4 optional unit

HSC410c Advocate for, and with, individuals, families, carers, groups and communities.

Mental Health Standards

A4.1 + 4.2 Promote effective communication and relationships.

A6.1, 6.2, 6.3 Promote effective communication where there are communication differences.

F1.1, 1.2, 1.3 Prepare, implement and evaluate agreed therapeutic group activities.

F3.1, 3.2, 3.3, 3.4 Prepare and provide agreed individual development activities.

G1.1, 1.2, 1.3 Establish, sustain and disengage from relationships with clients.

G12.1, 12.2 Represent individuals' interests when they are not able to do so themselves.

G13.1 Promote people's rights to make informed choices.

H4.1, 4.2 Support people in relation to personal and social interactions and environmental factors.

Further reading and references

Argyle, M. (1967) *The Psychology of Interpersonal Behaviour*. Harmondsworth: Penguin.
This is an excellent introduction to social psychology and it is very readable, deservedly a classic.

Babins, L. (1986) 'A humanistic approach to old-old people: A general model.' In *Activities, Adaptation and Aging*. New York: Haworth Press.

Goudie, F. and Stokes, G. (eds) (1990) *Working with Dementia*. Bicester: Speechmark/Winslow.

Jenkinson, B. (1992) 'Does reality orientation work?' *Nursing Times*. 13 May 88 (20) 39–40.

Kitwood, T. and Bredin, K. (1991) *Person to Person: A Guide to the Care of Those with Failing Mental Powers.* Second edition. Loughton: Gale Publications.

O'Donovan, S. (1996) 'A validation approach to severely demented clients.' *Nursing Standard 11*, 13–14, 48–52.

Rogers, C. (1951) *Client-Centred Therapy*. London: Constable.
This outlines Roger's counselling and helping skills and attitudes.

Rogers, C. (1961) *On Becoming a Person*. London: Constable.
This is worth a read if you are seeking to reflect upon your own life and helping skills. A classic in terms of both personal and professional aspects of life.

Williams, C. and Tappen, R. (1999) 'Can we create a therapeutic relationship with nursing home residents in the later stages of Alzheimer's disease.' *Journal of Psychosocial Nursing, 37*, 3, 28–34.

✔

Exercise 8.1

COMMUNICATION

In the following scenarios try to identify the feelings being expressed and what the hidden messages or reasons might be. Also assume that all the clients are in the latter stages of a dementia and that RO is no longer appropriate. Discuss how inappropriate the given response is and the effect it might have on the client. Finally, come up with a validation or resolution response and describe the positive effect you are hoping such a response will have.

Gladys
A client you are trying to feed is pushing you away shouting, 'It's poison, it's poison'. The nurse says, 'It's all right Gladys, it's from the kitchens. Look, Jim's eating it'.

Jim
Jim is found banging on the windows, crying and looking down the road. His wife has just left after her weekly visit. A carer comes up to Jim, puts her arms around him and says, 'It's OK Jim, she'll be back in a minute'.

Jean
Jean is sitting on the floor in a corner in tears, moaning and wailing incomprehensibly. She is clearly quite distressed. Two nurses try to pick her up saying, 'Come come Jean, we can't be having this. It'll all be all right. Come and have a cup of tea'.

Joan
Joan, aged 82, is in a nursing home. She is attempting to get out of the front door and, as you try and tempt her away with the promise of a cup of tea, she shouts, 'Let me go, it's late, she'll be worried. Where am I?' The nurse comes up to her and says, 'No Joan, it's fine, you live with us now'.

Chapter 9

Reminiscence

Key messages

- Reminiscence is both social and therapeutic and can be done in groups or on a one-to-one basis.
- It has many benefits for clients but also helps staff to get to know clients as individuals and thus promotes a person centred approach to care.

Most of us reminisce and reflect upon past experience more frequently than we think. We reflect upon past experience to guide present decision making, but more commonly we reminisce together socially by recounting both recent and distant past experiences shared. This gives us a sense of togetherness and a shared identity. Reminiscence is a very important aspect of working with all older people, but it can be especially useful with clients suffering dementia, because of their failing memories and urgent need to retain a sense of who they are. It involves looking back upon clients' lives and the experiences of their generation. Doing reminiscence work with clients also enables us to gain a better understanding of them as individuals. As we learn about their unique past we come to understand their needs that much better and we can then individualise the care we give them. We can take account of their preferences, likes, values and beliefs, which are unearthed through the reminiscence work.

The activity itself can boost self-esteem as the client is the expert in their own life and will enjoy telling carers and others about themselves and their achievements. Reminiscence work can be undertaken on a one-to-one basis or in groups which are useful in giving a sense of belonging, sharing common experiences and generating social interaction. Such sessions will usually become popular social events in their own right and can become a regular weekly event which clients look forward to.

There are many good reasons for taking the time and effort to bother with reminiscence work and these are outlined in this chapter.

Understanding

Listening to clients relive their lives through reminiscence can radically change our perception of them and will give us a far better understanding of them as individuals. We get a much more detailed insight into their personalities, values, beliefs and uniqueness just by listening to their stories. Such an insight allows us to better understand their needs and their behaviours. Reminiscence is doubly important if our clients suffer dementia, as the fund of information they can share with us is likely to be diminished and to lessen as time goes by. Thus we need to tap into it as soon as possible.

In a residential or nursing-home setting it is important to get to know clients as individuals. This will allow you to individualise care and treat people according to their unique needs. You need a thorough history of their lives and significant events. This doesn't just mean getting to know what they like to wear or eat; it means gaining an insight into every aspect of their being and past to find out their many other preferences and beliefs. You are trying to build up a picture of what is important to them, what makes them tick. Reminiscence can help you to build up a comprehensive biography, including work, school and family life, and so on, and thus an understanding of the client to which you can refer in your daily interactions and in so doing ensure that you tailor your care to those needs, preferences and beliefs. You need to end up with a sense of what was important to the client.

Reminiscence helps clients with dementia retain some sense of individuality. As their short-term memory declines, they increasingly inhabit the world of the long-term memory. It is essential that the carer explore this world in order to try to understand the client's needs and behaviour and see the world from their perspective. Gaining such an understanding can put meaning to otherwise unusual behaviour and speech. What was previously seen as problematic behaviour can be seen as a realistic way of coping.

Reminiscence also allows us to uncover significant personal events and anniversary dates which can form the focus of further reminiscence work with individuals and become a focus for annual celebrations. Using reminiscence as a guide to getting to know our clients as individuals we can eradicate much of the monotony and impersonal routine of institutional life. We all retain our individuality and uniqueness by recalling and sharing our pasts and by enabling the client to do this they can once again become the shop steward, the county champion hurdler, the young mother; in other words, an individual with a unique past, not just a client. Engaging in reminiscence with clients is also a very good way of building up relationships with them.

Belonging

The sharing of reminiscences is a social event. Whilst our own unique history sets us all apart as individuals, it also brings people of the same generation together since they have shared many common experiences and thus have a collective identity with a historical period. This experience, however, might vary radically from one individual to another and the experience, appreciation and memory of it will also vary. There are also many diverse groups and opinions within each generation. This plethora of cultural diversity, however, occurs within a certain historical time frame and it is this which can be identified with to give a sense of belonging. This sense of belonging, if achieved, can help remove the sense of isolation that old age and institutionalisation can bring.

Self-esteem

The clients are the custodians of the information in reminiscence. They have the facts and the lived experience about their generation and history and it is a great boost to the client's self-esteem if they are listened to, notice is taken of them and they are to be the expert. Roles are reversed: carers receive wisdom and information from clients, clients now cater for the carers' needs, the client becomes the giver and the carer the receiver. It is also very therapeutic for clients to listen to other clients giving similar accounts which validate their own. This confirms a sense of belonging and shared identity and, in doing so, again boosts self-esteem. Such sharing of reminiscences becomes crucial within institutional settings. It is easy, when in care, to become isolated, to feel remote and basically to feel as if you don't belong. Reminiscence work can help to combat this and give clients back a sense of belonging and identity.

Social skills

Engaging in reminiscence groups encourages sociability via the act of sharing and in so doing it also helps to maintain social skills. Quiet clients who do not normally join in can often be stimulated to air their own recollections in such groups. Being listened to by others will help build confidence in those who are normally quiet, reserved or shy. In order to enhance this function of reminiscence work, try making the sessions more of a special event, with cakes and tea.

Activity

It is sadly still the case that in many residential settings activity levels are woefully low. Running a reminiscence group is a therapeutic and easy way to combat such inactivity. Reminiscence is often also a springboard to discovering other interests and ideas which can form the basis of trips, outings and other activities worth trying. It can also give carers insight into interests clients once had, which they can try and revive. Increases in activity levels will usually also see a decrease in boredom and what is often perceived as 'disruptive' behaviour.

Life review

Reminiscence can be used as an opportunity to take stock of one's life and achievements. The process of looking back and putting things into perspective is common to us all at times. It is natural, as we get older, to want to re-examine past events and achievements. In reminiscence groups clients can examine how they used to cope and perhaps how they have succeeded against the odds. As carers we should try and ensure that reminiscence emphasises the positive. There is a danger that reminiscence could lead to feelings of sadness if a happy past is contrasted with bleak present. It is important that we focus on ability and achievement and project that into the present.

Resolution

Reminiscence can have important psychological benefits. If something from a client's past is bothering them and stopping them enjoying their life it needs to be resolved. One way of doing this is by talking it through in an attempt to resolve it. Sometimes there is no easy resolution and we have to learn to live with it, but often we need help to come to this conclusion. Often people can dwell on problems for long periods, because they are hard to face and resolve. Skilled reminiscence can be of great value here.

Clients should not be forced to raise difficult issues, but reminiscence can provide them with the opportunity to explore that which they would otherwise dwell on in sadness. However, some things can't be resolved easily and we should be wary of prolonging or increasing the sense of sadness felt and be mindful that occasionally the client may need skilled counselling if unresolved dilemmas are holding him back or causing distress. You might need to refer on to specialist help in such cases.

Reality Orientation

Retaining a sense of 'who I am' is important in dementia. Skilled one-to-one reminiscence can help a sufferer retain a sense of identity and individuality. Exploring your personal history helps retain a sense of uniqueness. One excellent way of undertaking reminiscence work with clients is to build up a scrapbook of the client's life, a sort of 'This is Your Life' as described earlier (see Exercise 9.1, p.91). It can include photographs, certificates, cuttings, membership cards, souvenirs, mementos and pictures of anything the client enjoyed, such as their favourite football team or a pet. Ask friends and relatives to build up the picture of the client's life, family, jobs, hobbies, holidays etc: what they enjoyed and what made them tick! The family will be grateful for the opportunity to celebrate the life of their loved one and to feel that they are participating in their care. Such a scrapbook will enable the carer to spend time with the client just sitting together and looking through it, chatting about the client's life and times. Producing such a scrapbook is also an opportunity for the client to feel empowered. Make it their project so that they can enjoy ownership.

Life story books

Life story books are really an extension of the scrapbook idea. First a time line of the client's life is worked out with the help of the client and relatives. This highlights significant milestones and achievements, both good times and bad times. Information is then gathered in more detail from one-to-one reminiscence sessions and relatives. A tape recorder can be used to aid gathering and remembering the material. This is written down as the text of the life story book, using the client's own words where possible. It is then supplemented with family photographs and mementos such as membership cards, postcards and relevant pictures from magazines. The result is a detailed insight into the client's life. The value of this, apart from the social and reminiscence value of making it, is that it provides a focus for interaction, conversation and ongoing reminiscence and identity work with the client. It is something that can be picked up, looked at and shared time and time again. It also enables carers to really get to know clients as individuals with unique histories. In doing so care patterns and practices can be altered to take account of that individuality. Choices relevant to the client can be offered in many aspects of daily living, the need for which was not apparent before.

Fun

A major reason for undertaking any activity is to have fun. If it is not fun then you are doing it wrong. We must be careful to ensure that clients wish to reminisce. Reminiscences are not necessarily the accurate recall of the facts, they are often more of a reinterpretation, after we have filtered out, either consciously or otherwise, that which we don't wish to remember. Recollections often give a rosier picture of the past, the so-called 'good old days'. There will be those who do not wish to reminisce, for their own good reasons, and this should be respected. The Second World War, for example, is often a focus for reminiscence because it had a huge impact upon the generation who lived through it. However, there will be many who do not wish to be reminded about what was, for them, a time of immense tragedy.

How to do it!

There is no one way of doing reminiscence work. You must adapt to the needs of the clients you are working with. There are obvious categories upon which to concentrate. The rich and famous are often a focus for reminiscence work but it is ordinary life, the 'humdrum' which makes up the greater part of our lives and this should be our major focus. It is work, school, family life and personal events which made us what we are. These are the things we have a shared experience of. Television personalities, sports stars and royalty have little real impact on our own lives, but that feeling on Christmas Eve when you are six is still with most of us.

Some research will be needed to explore clients' lives in detail. You might also explore local history. Some time and effort should go into finding trigger materials such as large pictures or, better still, actual objects and other memorabilia.

Groupwork

The great benefit from groupwork is the sharing it fosters and the opportunity it gives for practising social skills. General guidance is to keep groups small as this will ensure all get a chance to join in. Use plenty of props and triggers, such as pictures and objects to pass around. One excellent idea for any reminiscence theme is to make a group collage from magazine pictures. As has been mentioned previously, such sharing enhances self-esteem and feelings of belonging. Another advantage of groups is that they give you access to more memories. A good idea, linked to traditions of oral history being passed down the generations, is to organise some sessions with local schoolchildren. The children can learn about the past from primary sources and living experts, while the clients will benefit from the children probing and enhancing recall by asking pertinent – or impertinent – questions! Such sessions help to preserve cultural heritage and every client should be encouraged to feel they have valid stories to tell. It is important to remember though, that for some an individual approach is more suitable, especially where cognitive impairment is present.

Reminiscence in dementia

We have already mentioned that reminiscence is important in the early stages of dementia in retaining a sense of 'who I am'. Where cognitive ability is in decline it is very important to pitch it at the right level. Beware of creating anxiety in the early stages of dementia by using therapy which serves merely to emphasise the client's failing cognitive ability and memory. With the wrong client, reminiscence can be devastating and frightening. Similarly, in the later stages, do not enforce failure by trying to focus on the irretrievable. Do whatever leads to a happy outcome. Use plenty of props such as large pictures and things to handle. Have only one subject per session, so as not to confuse. Ensure you have a quiet, undisturbed environment. Know your client's unique histories and tailor the sessions to these.

When doing one-to-one work consider the compilation of 'bed boards': personal history and identity boards with photos of the client and their family, and mementos of the individual's life such as membership cards, pictures of favourite places, football teams, etc. A major benefit of reminiscence in dementia is that you are focusing on the long-term memory. In doing so you are giving the client the opportunity to be successful. They are listened to and given attention, valued for their expertise, and they receive a boost to their self-esteem (see the photocopiable major reminiscence themes resource on p.91).

Triggers

Below are just a few ideas for discussion themes and triggers.

The home and homelife

Everything domestic can come into this category, from washing socks to taking the rubbish out, and what people throw away today compared with a few years ago. Try to find some old photographs, old money, kitchen equipment, a darning toadstool, mothballs and other props. Other ideas are the street you lived in, what your house was like, bath time, bedtime, courtship, marriage, morals, child-birth, illness, old medicines, shaving equipment, family photos, Sunday lunch, church and religion, cookery books, entertainment in the evenings, knitting patterns and weekends.

Childhood

Discuss grandparents, siblings and other relatives clients can remember. Who were their best friends? What rhymes and games can they remember? Try and have some old toys or pictures of them to generate discussion and jog memories. Also try and get hold of some old sweets to taste, cigarette cards, old football boots and old annuals or comics. What street games did they play? What comics or books did they read? Other ideas for discussion are comics, sweets such as sherbert and liquorice, what clients did on wet days and at weekends, punish-ment, Christmas, pocket money, dolls, scrapbooks, dinky cars, marbles and conkers, Action Man, badges, playing cards. This list is short: get together with colleagues and come up with a much longer version adapted to your local area.

School

Ask how people used to get to school and discuss classrooms and teachers. Can clients remember their first day at school? What was their favourite and worst lesson? Discuss games, PE and sports day, school uniform, playtimes, school dinners, detention and other punishments. Again this list is short. Enlarge it with colleagues and clients. Try and borrow some old textbooks and chalk boards from the local museum, maybe a cane! Ask the local school if you can borrow some modern items to contrast with the old.

Work

Ask clients about their first jobs, the pay and conditions. Have some old photographs which can be passed around. Discuss unions, strikes and unemployment, holidays, pay slips and hours of work. Discuss what tools of the trade clients worked with and also enquire into breaks and lunches. A good idea is to cut out some modern job advertisements from a newspaper and discuss the wages and conditions now as compared to years ago. It might be possible to find some old pay packets, union cards, job advertisements and old tools.

Clothes

Try and find some old clothes to hand around or get some pictures of some such as long johns or petticoats. Other ideas for discussion topics are Sunday best, moth balls, cast-offs and hand-me-downs, shoes and underwear. If you can find any, have some old items of clothing such as a hat and cap, a petticoat or stockings to pass around. Remembering that fun is an essential factor, enquire as to the modern merits of thongs and mini skirts and men without shirts in public places! Have some cuttings of modern clothes or the real thing to pass around and contrast these with. Hats, jewellery, buttons, sewing equipment and shoes can all be discussed. Ask the group what they think of tattoos and body jewellery!

Housework

Topics might include cleaning, wash day, carpets, rugs, appliances, vacuum cleaners, men and housework, irons, getting clothes dry, doing the washing, shopping, mangles, washing the dishes, carbolic soap, launderettes, polishing, dusting. Ask clients about decorating and moving house: these two topics will provide much material for discussion. A trawl around a good car boot sale will get you some useful props such as an old iron and an old sewing machine.

Physical triggers

Try to build up a resource of triggers such as pictures cut from magazines, objects to handle, tape recordings etc. Actually showing a client an image will trigger more memories than if you merely describe it or talk about it. Letting the client see the object in the flesh, hold it, and use it, will spark off even more memories. Have a look around your local antiques shops and boot fairs for old household equipment and old annuals etc. Go to your local museum custodian and librarian and get in contact with local clubs and societies. These should be able to provide you with a range of trigger material and possibly visiting speakers.

Remember, triggers should encompass all the senses, sight and hearing are obvious, but touch is equally important, as are smell and taste. Bearing this in mind will increase the range of triggers you might consider using. Scents, textures and tastes can provide an interesting and stimulating session. The tactile stimulation of using real old props and artefacts is important; there is nothing like holding the real thing in your hands again. This will encourage demonstration: 'No, we did it like this!' Be creative and hold reminiscence cookery and baking sessions, using the old recipes and methods. This could be followed by a tasting or it could be a good excuse for a tea dance. A large bar of carbolic soap will be good to handle and smell and the senses will trigger more memories than just the mention of carbolic soap. Peeling potatoes would be another good idea for triggering memories and seeing who has still got the 'knack'.

With regard to auditory triggers, it is said that it is impossible to separate a sound from its visual image. This being so, music is especially good at evoking memories. Try getting hold of or recording your own sounds such as children at play or the bustle of a busy train station. Check the local newspapers as they often have a 'Yesteryear' section, which can be read aloud to allow opportunity for reminiscence. Go through all your magazines in a group with clients before you throw them out. Collect pictures of places, people, objects and anything the clients find interesting. Collate these into scrapbooks with themes such as places, wildlife, people, etc. This is an activity in itself. Once finished, the scrapbooks are useful for just sitting with a client looking at it and chatting. They are an excellent dementia care resource, as just sitting looking at pictures together demonstrates your message that you like being with the client. The emphasis is on interaction and client involvement, so don't show long videos, just quick snapshots to generate discussion. Good historical videos can be watched together on another occasion.

Health and Social Care National Occupational Standards

This chapter relates to many of the induction and foundation standards but in particular to the following level standards:

Level 2 core units

HSC21 a, b + c Communicate with and complete records for individuals.

Level 2 optional units

HSC210 a, b + c Support individuals to access and participate in recreational activities.
HSC212 a, b + c Support individuals during therapy sessions.

Level 3 core units

HSC31 a, b + c Promote effective communication for and about individuals.

Level 3 optional units

> HSC332 a, b + c Support the social, emotional and identity needs of individuals.
>
> HSC369 a, b + c Support individuals with specific communication needs.
>
> HSC393 a, b + c Prepare, implement and evaluate agreed therapeutic group activities.

Mental Health Standards

> F1.1, 1.2, 1.3 Prepare, implement and evaluate agreed therapeutic group activities.
>
> F3.1, 3.2, 3.3, 3.4 Prepare and provide agreed individual development activities.
>
> G9.1, 9.2 Enable people to choose and participate in activities which are meaningful to them.

Further reading and references

Jones, G. and Meisen, B. (1992) *Care Giving in Dementia: Research and Applications.* London: Routledge.

Exercise 9.1

PERSONAL SCRAPBOOK

- As an exercise try making a scrapbook of things related to your own history and interests. Have a look at the self-assessment you carried out upon yourself in Exercise 6.12 (p.58) and use this as a starting point.

- Fill the scrapbook with mementos and pictures of the things that are or were important to you over the years.

- Bear in mind what you would want people to talk to you about if you should begin to lose a sense of who you are as a result of a dementia-type illness and needed to be looked after by people who did not know you before your illness.

- What pictures, documents or other material need to go in there for others to get a good idea about you?

This will be an interesting thing for you to do for yourself but, when it is finished, to make it harder and to emphasise the need to get to know what is most important to our clients, you now have only a sheet of paper. Select those pictures which are so important that they cannot be missed and make a poster of what's important to you.

Exercise 9.2

MAJOR REMINISCENCE THEMES RESOURCE

Work, shopping, gardening, school, church, family life, hobbies, wild flowers, entertainment, royalty, the seasons, cricket, tennis, food, countryside, the pub, military service, zoos, London, wildlife, childhood, towns lived in, seaside holidays, famous people, gardening, shopping, household chores, farms, town life, transport, music, women's role, hiking, villages, places, castles, stately homes, pets, fairground rides, toys, sport, antiques, everyday household objects, art, occupations, cooking, Christmas, birthdays, special occasions such as Halloween, weather, clothes and fashion.

The hiking and zoos are from my personal list. You need to find out what would be on your clients' personal lists. Write your own personal list of themes to see what other possibilities there are: football, dogs, etc.

Chapter 10

Independence and Good Practice

Key messages

- Independence is often eroded by carers' assumptions about lack of ability.
- The focus of care needs to be on giving back roles and responsibilities rather than taking them over.
- Lack of time is not an excuse to deskill a client.

Dementia can bring about loss of independence simply via stereotyping. To the lay person the label of dementia brings with it powerful assumptions that sufferers will be unable to do much for themselves, be unable to communicate and need almost complete care. Even as carers we can on occasion tend towards this view and make assumptions about a person's ability or lack of it. We tend not to take risks, we tend to stick to routines and may do things for clients instead of with them, or allowing them the time to do it for themselves (see Exercise 10.1, p.92).

Good practice guidelines

In dementia care it is important that people maintain their independence for as long as possible. Below are good practice guidelines which can help with that goal.

Slow down

It is important that people are encouraged to do as much for themselves as possible. The pace and delivery of much institutional care can erode opportunities for self-care and hence the maintenance of skills. Allowing people to do things for themselves allows them to feel successful and for their confidence to be maintained. When staff begin to intervene in order to speed things up, by helping a person to get dressed or to eat, they are eroding those abilities alongside the client's confidence and self-esteem. Carers must slow down and allow time for clients to succeed.

Daily living skills

A key focus in maintaining independence should be the normal activities of living, such as dressing, washing and eating etc. These self-care skills are the important ones which make us truly independent. However, there are many other aspects of ordinary life, such as meal preparation and shopping, in which clients should be included. These will be explored further in Chapter 27 on normalisation.

Prompting

The client should be guided with minimal prompting and given time to ensure that they are allowed to succeed. This is a skilled intervention and requires that you know your client well. Too much help will deskill your clients and erode their confidence, too little can also bring on feelings of failure if they are left to flounder. Verbally describing the next step to take in a sequence of events will often be sufficient. Miming the actions is another very powerful tool as you demonstrate what is needed, providing a visual clue. It may be that you can initiate the act, guide the client and then let them continue with it. Often this is all that is needed to trigger the memory of the next step. Where more prompting is necessary you can often begin to do it and then let them carry on or at least finish it off, so that they have taken some part in it. Remember that good prompting will rely on the communication skills described earlier.

Routine

It is helpful to clients if they stick to a familiar routine and thus know what activity follows another in the day. The client will usually have a personal sequence of doing things and they must be allowed to adhere to this rather than be forced to fit the institutional timetable of events. Such a familiar routine can help prolong orientation to time and offset some of the other creeping uncertainties which a dementia can bring. Carers need to elicit from relatives what the client's previous routines and preferences were, this will include morning and evening routines as well as mealtimes, drink breaks, walks etc. It might also include very detailed preferences, such as when exactly a client likes to brush their teeth, or do they get dressed first or use the toilet first when they get up? Establishing or consolidating the client's daily routine will go a long way towards helping them to remain independent. Taking this to its logical next step, the client may well have routines for different days of the week, which can be adhered to. This might incorporate having a lie-in at the weekends, shopping on a particular day, doing laundry on another particular day, a different Sunday and Saturday routine. Again, relatives will be able to help you to find out more.

Realistic and achievable

Clients should be encouraged to participate in activities that are both realistic and achievable. Success in such activities will help to boost confidence and so foster independence. Many activities, such as games and crafts, can be adapted to give a sense of personal achievement and success. Being engaged in activity will enable the client to feel useful and wanted and there are many activities around the home and garden that any client can do: drying and sorting out cutlery, tidying magazines or books, dusting, cleaning, sweeping the path. These tasks and many more can give a client a feeling of achievement and independence. They are also an opportunity for shared activity and relationship building. End results are not important, just the client's sense of accomplishment and self-worth.

Praise

Praise should be given to recognise success, and even the smallest efforts and gains should be thus rewarded. Remember to show praise non-verbally with smiles and touch as these are powerful reinforcers and will be recognised when verbal praise cannot be understood.

Appliances

Often skills of dexterity can be lost and it is helpful to use aids and adaptations in order to maintain independence. Swapping a plate for a dish and using a non-slip place mat, for example, can make the difference between someone feeding themselves or having to be fed. There are many excellent ideas such as adapted cups and cutlery, grab rails for baths, etc. Velcro for clothing is also excellent and can help maintain someone's ability to both dress and toilet.

Reality Orientation

RO has already been discussed and it is important here to remind us of its role in maintaining independence through the use of signs, notices and picture clues on doors and drawers. A large clock and orientation board giving daily details are also important in allowing people to reorient themselves rather than having to ask. Remember also that continual verbal RO will help.

Health and Social Care National Occupational Standards

This chapter relates to many of the induction and foundation standards but in particular to the following level standards:

Level 2 core units

HSC24 a Relate to and support individuals in the way they choose.

Level 2 optional units

HSC211 a, b + c Support individuals to take part in developmental activities.

Level 3 core units

HSc35a Develop supportive relationships that promote choice and independence.

Level 3 optional

HSC332 a, b + c Support the social, emotional and identity needs of individuals.

HSC 3116 a, b + c Contribute to a culture that values and respects the diversity of individuals.

Mental Health Standards

A3.1, 3.2, 3.3 Promote the values and principles underpinning best practice.

D4.1 Identify individuals' needs and circumstances.

G 8.1, 8.2 Enable people to identify and address their personal spiritual needs.

G11.1, 11.2, 11.3 Promote the social inclusion of people with mental health needs.

G13.1 Promote people's rights to make informed choices.

M3.1, 3.2, 3.3 Contribute to developing and maintaining cultures and strategies in which people are respected and valued as individuals.

O9.1, 9.2, 9.3 Promote people's equality and respect for diversity.

Care Homes for Older People: National Minimum Standards

7.1 to 7.6 These are concerned with each service user having a unique plan of care which is reviewed monthly and covers health, personal and social needs.

14.1 to 14.5 Relate to maintaining autonomy, choice and personal control.

Further reading and references

Holden, U. and Woods, R.T. (1995) *Positive Approaches to Dementia Care*. Edinburgh: Churchill Livingstone.

Phair, L. and Good, V. (1995) *Dementia: A Positive Approach*. London: Scutari Press.

✓

Exercise 10.1

REGAINING ROLES AND INDEPENDENCE

- For each client, list everything you do for them.

- Examine whether all of these are really necessary.

- List what clients can do for themselves.

- Think of ways you can use these preserved skills to increase the range of things they can do for themselves.

- Invent jobs for them to do which use these skills.

- What aspects of *your* job can clients help you with?

Exercise 10.2

DIGNITY AND PRIVACY

- How does the illness of dementia erode a person's dignity?

- Think of times when the care you give might be an intrusion on dignity or privacy. List the aspects of institutional care that can erode dignity and privacy. Consider a typical client's day and go through all the interventions and interactions you might have with them, what you do with and for them.

- Draw up a list of ways you can change practice to better preserve dignity and privacy.

- Share this in a group discussion and iron out all the excuses as to why it might not happen. Brain storm what will get in the way of your good ideas, then brain storm ways around the blocks.

Exercise 10.3

DEINSTITUTIONALISATION

- What differences can you think of between caring for a family member at home and caring for a client in a nursing home?

- With colleagues, make a list of the things you would not be able to do because of the nursing home setting. Try and identify all the little things and special touches which are so important to us all which would not be possible in this setting. Consider the activities of daily living and the social and psychological aspects of care.

- Write these down on a flip chart.

- Having created your list, you can consider together ways of introducing those 'touches' into your care practice.

- Again, try to think of what will get in the way of doing this and think of ways to overcome these.

Chapter 11

Person Centred Care

Key messages
- Dementia does not strip the client of their personhood.
- Good care can give personhood to the client.

Personhood

This is what we are aiming to retain and foster in our clients, but what exactly is it? There are many different definitions in the literature but it can be broken down into the following core elements:

- Having social relationships.

- Being distinct; having identity.

- Being respected and acknowledged.

- Being able to act.

- Having feelings acknowledged.

- Having a sense of belonging.

People with dementia have lost the ability to preserve their own personhood and need carers to protect and promote it for them.

Value and worth

Institutional care can easily undermine one's sense of self-worth and confidence as one loses control over many areas of life.

Suffering from dementia does not mean that you cannot enjoy a happy life. In nursing homes it is the care worker who is key in ensuring that this happens. The starting point is in seeing the resident not as someone with dementia but as an individual person with a unique history. Chapter 6 on individualised care will show you how to achieve this. In addition to this there are some general principles which will help you to move towards a person centred approach in your care. Poor care can leave sufferers miserable and unhappy but, by adopting a person centred approach, we can go some considerable way to ensuring that our clients are happy, contented and retain their identity and personhood.

Recognition

Use every opportunity to acknowledge the person and that they exist. Always say their name. Create excuses to interact with them even if it is just for short periods of a few seconds or a minute. Use reminiscence and self-identity work such as life story books to help them to remain unique. Enhancing the sufferer's sense of individuality is a way of connecting with the person, not the illness. If we focus too much on the illness we can easily lose sight of the person. At its simplest, recognition is just about giving people some attention, making a conscious effort to break away from our many tasks and sharing some time with a client.

Give choice

Include clients in decisions; make sure you are aware of their preferences and give them the opportunities to make choices. Simple things like letting them choose a biscuit rather than giving them one are very important. The little things you do add up to a bigger picture of respect. You are treating them as persons not objects. The whole day is punctuated by decisions – what to wear, what to eat, what to do etc., the list is endless – so include the person in decisions affecting them. In this way you are moving away from treating people as unresponsive and incapable to regarding them as individuals in their own right.

> **Discussion point**
> How can you increase the range of choices offered to your clients in the average day? It might be helpful to look at each client in turn and try to come up with one improvement for each.

Stimulation

Provide the opportunity for activity. Make it possible for people to join in. As far as possible put the emphasis on you helping them rather than them helping you, so that clients have a sense of being in control. Participation in activity alongside the praise you give will foster confidence in the client's own abilities. Celebrate anything, not just birthdays and obvious occasions. Use anything as an excuse and focus on what the client enjoys. Make it a special event and an opportunity to boost clients' self-esteem by giving frequent praise and simply spending time with people having fun. Ignore mistakes and concentrate on the achievements, however small.

Being there

Archaeologists will understand the importance of the concept of 'being there' – they learn much about the lives of past peoples by being where they lived. Just being there is equally important in dementia care. Spend time with people, not just when you have a task to perform, but for the pleasure of being with them. Initiate social contact, as clients with dementia often cannot do this for themselves. The unconditional closeness you show will give people a sense of being valued and wanted. Listen to clients and try to gain a real insight into how they feel. Get physically close and give a sense of comfort and warmth. This is especially important in the later stages of dementia when verbal channels of communication are lost.

Respect

Preserve dignity by giving respect, such as always knocking on people's doors before entering. Always explain what you are doing and why, even if the person cannot understand you. Do not lie. This seems obvious but often it is tempting to tell a lie in order to avoid a situation we might find difficult to handle. Once we start evading the truth we begin to erode any trust the client has in us. Being honest and telling the truth gives the client a chance to make sense of their situation and to make choices about it. Honesty avoids us making their confusion worse. Always treat the person as an adult and do not patronise them. Again this sounds obvious but it is still common to come across an attitude which regards the client with dementia as childlike. All interactions and activities should be age appropriate so as to avoid insulting the dignity of clients.

Socialisation

Socialisation is extremely important, as we discussed in detail in Chapter 7. Suffice it to say here that social events provide the opportunity for interaction, for social skills to be maintained, for relationships to be developed and for having fun. In an institutional setting, social events are also good for fostering a sense of belonging. This is important when many previous associations have often been lost.

Validation

The validation approach entails accepting the client's version of reality rather than correcting it. It also means responding at every available opportunity to the emotions and feelings the client expresses. To ignore someone's feelings or expressed emotions, perhaps by using distraction when they are upset, is tantamount to saying that their feelings do not matter. Even where confusion is severe and you can't understand what is uttered, look for the hidden meanings in what is said and recognise the underlying feelings. By doing this you can validate those feelings and try to understand the world as the sufferer sees it.

A person centred approach to care will see the carer trying to gain an understanding of the client's world, to connect with it and to find meaning in otherwise meaningless speech and behaviour. You are striving for something closer to empathy than just sympathy, you try to get a feel for what it must really be like to be in the client's world.

Empowerment

Do not rush clients, don't try to take over – allow the person to do as much for themselves as they can, letting them set the pace. It is easier to do it for yourself sometimes, but try to allocate time for sufferers to do things for themselves. Inclusion and providing the opportunity to make decisions also empowers and gives the person a sense of having some control over their life. Do things *with* rather than *for* the person as this will foster a feeling of independence. Focus on retained abilities and provide the opportunity to display success. Seek out opportunities to give praise in order to help people feel valued and useful.

Inclusion

Be an enabler, create opportunities for the person to be included in the day-to-day things we take for granted. Look at all the activities of daily living, the running of the nursing home, activities, jobs etc. Explore the opportunities for involvement because doing this will give residents a sense of being useful and a sense of belonging. They can begin to feel they are a part of what is going on around them and begin to get a sense of being involved, taking part and running their own lives. Adapt the environment not the person, get carers involved, be creative, break the mould. See the Checklist of personhood friendly practices on p.106.

Conclusion

It is very demanding to be a carer – the financial rewards are little, the work care assistants do is not given sufficient recognition – but it can be very rewarding. At the end of the day caring is about giving the person respect and dignity, about fostering independence and giving people a sense of being wanted and valued as individuals. Often it is the little things in life which make a difference but which get overlooked in our busy work schedules. However, if anything can create a meaningful existence out of the bewilderment of confusion, if anything can create happiness where there was misery, it is the care worker.

Health and Social Care National Occupational Standards

This chapter relates to many of the induction and foundation standards but in particular to the following level standards:

Level 2 core units

HSC21b Listen to and respond to individuals' questions and concerns.

HSC24a Relate to and support individuals in the way they choose.

HSC27 a, b + c Support individuals in their daily living.

HSC210 a, b + c Support individuals to access and participate in recreational activities.

HSC211 a, b + c Support individuals to take part in developmental activities.

HSC218 a, b + c Support individuals with their personal care needs.

Level 2 optional units

HSC233 a + b Relate to and interact with individuals.

HSC234 a + b Ensure your own actions support the equality, diversity, rights and responsibilities of individuals.

Level 3 core units

HSC33 a + b Reflect on and develop your practice.

HSC35 a + b Promote choice and independence and respect the diversity and difference of individuals.

Level 3 optional units

HSC332 a, b + c Support the social, emotional and identity needs of the individual.

HSC334 a, b + c Provide a home and family environment for individuals.

HSC350 a, b + c Recognise, respect and support the spiritual well-being of individuals.

HSC3111 a + b Promote equality, diversity, rights and responsibilities of individuals.

HSC3116 a, b + c Contribute to promoting a culture that values and respects the diversity of individuals.

Level 4 core units

HSC43 a + b Take responsibility for the continuing professional development of self and others.

Level 4 optional units

HSC414 Assess individual needs and preferences.

Care Homes for Older People: National Minimum Standards

7.1 to 7.6 These standards relate to an individualised plan of care based on a comprehensive assessment to ensure individualised care.

10.3 Service users wear their own clothes at all times.

14.1 to 14.5 These standards relate to allowing clients to exercise choice and control over their lives.

Further reading and references

Crisp, J. (1999) 'Towards a partnership in maintaining personhood.' In T. Adams and C. Clarke (eds) *Dementia Care; Developing Partnerships in Practice*. Edinburgh: Churchill Livingstone.

This is a very good and essentially practical chapter looking at both the theory and practicality of fostering personhood. There are two essential messages underpinning the chapter and if all else is lost then just these two messages are worth hanging on to. First, the illness of dementia does not strip someone of their personhood. It is there, you just have to find it. Second, the most important truth and essential rule of caring (if only one thing is done this has to be it), is that care-giving behaviour can foster personhood. Good care can turn a subjectively horrendous dementia into a more tolerable, even happy, person centred experience.

Kitwood, T. and Bredin, K. (1991) *Person to Person: A Guide to the Care of Those with Failing Mental Powers.* Second edition. Loughton: Gale Publications.

✓

Exercise 11.1

PERSONHOOD: WHAT AND HOW?

Take each of the core elements (discussed on p.98) in turn and consider in a group what you understand by them. Try to think of ways in which you can facilitate each category.

Exercise 11.2

PERSONAL NEEDS

- With a group of colleagues, each write down a list of things you need in your life and what especially you need to make you feel good and happy.

- Share these and write them all down to come up with a joint list of key features.

- Now consider if you provide these things for your clients or whether they can experience them or have access to them.

- If not, why not?

- For each of the key features you have identified, discuss how you might be able to provide them.

Exercise 11.3

BEING VALUED

- Think about what it is to be valued ourselves.

- What do people do to make us feel valued and wanted?

- How can you help clients retain a sense of being valued, a sense of still being important?

Exercise 11.4

CHANGING ROUTINES

- Mealtimes are a perfect opportunity for interaction.

- How can you make changes to your mealtimes to foster interaction in your clients?

- Can you identify other daily routines which could be used to provide the opportunity for communication and interaction?

Exercise 11.5

EMPOWERMENT AND ROUTINE

- Think about your daily routines at work. Is there scope for change in a way that will empower clients?

- For each client think of one way in which they could do more for themselves.

Exercise 11.6

WHAT ARE YOUR NEEDS?

Discuss in a group what your personhood needs are and whether you meet similar needs in clients. If you do not, what action could be taken to ensure those needs are met in your work setting?

✔

Exercise 11.7

A CHECKLIST OF PERSONHOOD FRIENDLY PRACTICES

A (not exhaustive) list of positive acts and qualities which, if achieved, would lead to the nurturing of personhood.

- Be honest – don't lie – explain all you do.

- Empower, don't take over.

- Treat each person as an adult, an individual.

- Acknowledge their existence by inclusion and communication.

- Give attention.

- Recognise the person – use names and touch.

- Encourage – don't limit – find ways to include.

- Place a high value on social interaction – initiate social contact.

- Work together in shared tasks, jobs and activities.

- Show that you are listening.

- Create opportunities for interaction.

- Find abilities and strengths and interests.

- Avoid labelling.

- Let the person set the pace – allow time.

- Acknowledge and validate feelings and experience.

- Facilitate expression of feelings.

- Include people in everything.

- Listen for feelings behind words – even if the words are nonsensical.

- Learn their past.

- Be creative and ignore mistakes.

- Find reasons to give praise.

- Remind them of past achievements.

- Create opportunities to make choices.

- Consult with the person about preferences.

- Avoid too many questions.

- Change situations to avoid mistakes.

- Break routines to allow choice and inclusion.

- Encourage fun.

- Celebrate anything and everything.

- Relax, be near, sit together, hold hands.

- Respect wishes and values from past.

- Show pleasure in them and their actions.

- Adapt the environment not the person.

- Encourage carer and family involvement.

- Use the senses for shared enjoyment and communication.

- Break the mould.

Remember that the goal is to promote self-respect and self-esteem.

Dementia Care Training Manual for Staff Working in Nursing and Residential Settings © Danny Walsh 2006

Chapter 12

Bad Practice and Abuse

Key messages

- Bad practice and abuse are often very subtle.
- Exposing abuse can be hard and can make you unpopular with the abusers; but think if the victim was you or a member of your family – what would you want the carer to do?
- It is our duty to speak out and protect the vulnerable.

Recognising the signs of poor practice

Most carers have at some time worked in an area so bad as to make them wish that they never end up there. With colleagues generate a list of what it is exactly which makes these places so bad. What aspects of poor care lead to clients looking bored, anxious, withdrawn, apathetic and depressed? Once the list is generated, honestly appraise the care you collectively give and the quality of your clients' lives to see if there are any areas you could improve upon.

Recognising poor care is the key to eliminating it. Poor care is usually the result of ignorance and just not knowing how to do things better. This can be eliminated by training. Sometimes, however, it is because carers don't care and this is where it becomes abuse.

Malignant social psychology

This concept comes from the work of Tom Kitwood (1997). He argued that it is possible to be happy in a dementia and it is possible to be sad in a dementia. What makes the difference between the two is the care you receive. How we interact with people can turn their existence into a miserable or a happy one. Kitwood felt that poor care put clients under even more stress than they already had from coping with the dementia. This stress causes more neurological damage and thus makes the dementia worse. Kitwood identified certain behaviours that carers do which gives rise to stress and unhappiness. These make up what he calls 'malignant social psychology'.

Examples are:

- *Treachery* – Using lies or tricks to gain compliance or avoid awkward situations. Doing this usually means ignoring clients' feelings and is taking the easy way out. We should be honest, validate the client's experience and help them to talk about how they feel.

- *Disempowerment* – Not giving people the time to do things. Doing things for people that they can do themselves, usually to save ourselves time; for example, dressing or feeding them. Not giving them the assistance they need to succeed.

- *Infantilisation* – Treating people like children, patronising them. This can reinforce their feelings of uselessness. Clients are adults and need adult language and adult responses. Even though we often engage with clients at a simplistic level, using short sentences and repeating words, this is done in an adult manner.

- *Intimidation* – Using threats or power or just putting clients in situations where they feel anxious and uncertain. Such bad care is born of frustration and intolerance on the part of the carer. They are a form of abuse, making the client afraid and sad.

- *Labelling* – Focusing on the label, not the person; seeing only the dementia, thus setting up expectations of failure and treating everybody who has the label the same. A consequence of not knowing our clients as individuals.

- *Outpacing* – Deskilling to save time, failing to slow down so that the client can be included, speaking to fast so that the client can't understand.

- *Invalidation* – Ignoring the client's feelings and their reality. Even though we might not be able to communicate verbally with clients we can still recognise the emotions they display and thus their feelings. We have a duty to validate these. Likewise, the duty exists to validate whatever reality the client is living in. Invalidation ignores the client's reality and feelings. They are left wondering why no one cares, feeling isolated and more lost and afraid than ever. Yet it is easy to share laughter and to comfort someone by putting your arms around them. These simple human actions show the person that you care for and value them.

- *Banishment* – Excluding people because of behaviour or diagnosis. Exclusion may take the form of physical isolation, such as putting someone in another room, or social isolation, by not including them.

- *Objectification* – Treating as an object not a real person, or as if they were not there. Clients look bored, anxious, withdrawn, apathetic and depressed.

- *Ignoring* – Carrying on and talking about people as if they were not there. Ignoring clients is giving them the message that they are not important, not worth bothering with. It confirms their realisation that they are apart from life; it confirms their growing feelings of isolation and insecurity.

- *Denying choice* – Not giving the opportunity to choose. Imposing your will. There are many choices clients can be offered in many of the different aspects of daily living.

- *Denying attention* – Not engaging with the client. Not giving them your time, even for small periods. Not calling them by name. Denying attention to clients who are obviously in need of it. Being too busy is used as an excuse to give time and reassurance.

- *Medication* – Sometimes this is used as a management tool. Problem behaviour is all too frequently managed by sedation rather than a real attempt to understand the root cause of it and deal with it.

- *Denying stimulation* – Leaving clients unstimulated and doing nothing for large periods of time. Understaffing and poor care often leads to whole groups of clients being left in a room with the television on.

- *Accusation* – The person is blamed for the results of their dementia, for example if they spill something, are slow or get something wrong. In doing so we are almost telling the client they are worthless or at best a nuisance. The individual is likely to be more upset than us at their errors and failing abilities. Blame arises out of intolerance and a lack of understanding of the dementia, but it induces fear, depression and sadness.

Often problem behaviours can arise as a response to poor care and malignant social psychology. Such problems can be overcome when more positive approaches are adopted. If clients are struggling with their dementia and in understanding what is going on around them, they will be feeling vulnerable. If they are then treated in an uncaring way their fears and anxieties will be greatly increased at the point where they need most support and reassurance. The result is likely to be behaviours which we then classify as problematic.

Abuse

Abuse is…making the lives of clients miserable. This is probably the most important part of the book. If you see abuse, report it and put an end to it, you have done a very good thing. Yet all too often carers are reluctant and scared to report abuse for fear of losing their jobs or upsetting others they have to work with. Abuse is performed by bullies, and where it occurs it is likely that carers are being bullied too. It is difficult being on your own and going out on a limb, but you have a duty of care. Exposing abuse is easier if you have an ally or allies, so gather your evidence and get others to back you up and expose it. Write things down as soon after the event(s) as possible so that your account is accurate and credible. Describe the incident(s) of poor care and make a note of times, dates and people. Think of it as happening to your parents or children, be angry and defend your clients.

Our client group is particularly vulnerable. They often cannot complain or explain how they feel. So we must be extra vigilant in our observation and advocacy. Abuse can happen in any setting from the client's own home, to day care and residential, nursing home and hospital settings. Clients whose dementia features aggression are likely to be at greater risk of abuse through retaliation and carers' frustration, which arise from a paucity of support services.

What is abuse?

Abuse takes many forms. Some are obvious, such as hitting and slapping and re-straining, but some may be quite subtle, such as overuse of medication or forms of psychological abuse such as ignoring and humiliation. Other forms of abuse are sexual abuse, emotional abuse, blaming, threats, neglect, enforced isolation, inactivity, discrimination, financial abuse and denial of privacy and respect, food, warmth, clothing, etc. In institutions abuse may arise out of not allowing them choices or preferences, or by subjecting them to a routine not in keeping with their prior lifestyle, cultural or other beliefs.

The general paucity of services to help people looking after relatives with dementia at home is a large factor in fuelling much abuse in community settings. Because of this we must add society itself to the list of abusers. There is generally a low level of priority given to dementia care and this has been the pattern for many years. Ageism is rife and resources to support clients with dementia have to compete with many other worthy causes. The evidence suggests that 'society' is abusing carers too by denying them adequate levels of support. The withdrawal of the NHS from respite care has added to carer strain since the only alternative is costly, private care.

Institutionalisation

Rigid adherence to one routine and denial of an individualised approach could itself be said to be a form of abuse (see Exercise 12.3, p.115). If we tried to enforce one religion and only catered for the needs of one cultural group we would be open to claims of abuse by neglect of individual needs.

Factors likely to make matters worse

- Lack of training.

- Low staff morale.

- Poor supervision/support.

- Low pay.

- Low status of care work.

- Poor staffing levels.

- Reliance on agency staff.

- Poor management.

- Poor support in a crisis.

- Lack of staff meetings.

- Lack of individualised approach to care.

- Seeing all clients as demented rather than individuals with a dementia.

- Low levels of involvement of care assistants in case discussions and key working.

Inactivity

Abuse comes in many forms and can be quite subtle and often hard to detect or prove. One of its less obvious but extremely common forms, is inactivity. Often the hotel aspects of care, are very good – good food, nice décor, etc. – and physical aspects of care, such as hygiene, are also good. But all too often psychological needs are left unmet and clients are left sitting around all day long doing nothing. This is abuse. It exacerbates sensory deprivation, depression, disorientation, dependency and cognitive decline. Try it. Try being a client for a day. Agree with your manager to spend the day as a client, waking to sleeping. In the experience you are not allowed to watch television at all. Dementia would most likely reduce the television to a bizarre, not understandable background noise, so you can't use it to ease your day as a client. Report back your experiences to the staff group.

Health and Social Care National Occupational Standards

This chapter relates to many of the induction and foundation standards but in particular to the following level standards:

Level 2 core units

HSC24b Treat people with respect and dignity.

HSC24c Assist in the protection of individuals.

Level 2 optional units

HSC226a Identify aspects of individuals' lives that may cause distress.

HSC234a Respect the rights and interests of individuals.

HSC240 a, b + c Contribute to the identification of the risk of danger (and abuse) to individuals and others.

Level 3 optional units

HSC332b Support individuals to develop and maintain self-esteem and a positive self-image.

HSC335 a, b + c Contribute to the protection of individuals from harm and abuse.

HSC395 a, b + c Contribute to assessing and act upon risk of danger, harm and abuse.

HSC3111 a Promote the rights and interests of individuals.

Mental Health Standards

D4.2 Identify the risk of abuse, failure to protect and harm to self and others in accordance with relevant legislation.

G12.1, 12.2 Represent individuals' interests when they are not able to do so themselves.

G13.1 Promote people's rights to make informed choices.

J4.1, 4.2, 4.3 Contribute to the protection of individuals from abuse.

O9.1, 9.2, 9.3 Promote people's equality and respect for diversity.

Care Homes for Older People: National Minimum Standards

10.1 to 10.7 All of these standards centre on aspects of privacy and dignity and the avoidance of bad practice. They cover personal care, hygiene needs, staff entering rooms, maintaining social contacts, wearing own clothes and respect.

12.1 to 12.4 These relate to leisure activity, mealtimes, religion, socialisation and choice.

13.1 to 13.6 These relate to involvement in the wider community, privacy with visitors and the absence of restrictions.

14.1 Maximising the client's capacity to exercise personal autonomy and choice.

18.1 to 18.6 These standards relate to the avoidance, reporting and procedures for dealing with physical, financial, material, psychological and sexual abuse alongside discrimination and degrading treatment, whether deliberate or through negligence or ignorance.

Further reading and references

Action on Elder Abuse website: www.elderabuse.org.uk

Kitwood, T. (1997) *Dementia Reconsidered: The Person Comes First.* Buckingham: Open University Press.

Penhale, B. (2003) 'Elder abuse and people with dementia.' In T. Adams and J. Manthorpe (eds), *Dementia Care.* London: Arnold.

✔

Exercise 12.1

NIGHTMARE!

- Imagine your worst nightmare of a nursing or residential home and brain storm a list of bad care that could occur.

- Try and recall all the bad practices you have witnessed when working elsewhere.

- Think about what relatives might complain about and what you would be angry about if it happened to your mother.

- Think about physical, social and psychological abuse and make lists of possible forms each of the abuses might take.

- Now think about how you can safeguard against it happening.

Exercise 12.2

SCENARIOS: ABUSE OR NOT?

For each scenario ask the questions: Is this abuse? If so, how could it be overcome? And what action should be taken?

1. Sheila wandered all the time and in doing so she interfered with other patients, touching them and pulling their hair. Relatives had complained so the ward decided to sit her so close to a table that she could not get up.

2. Kate was on the first placement of her nursing course, in a local nursing home. At the placement she witnessed a carer stopping a client with a walking frame from sitting down. The carer insisted that the client walk to her room and back because she said she had to have some exercise. The carer blocked the client's way as she tried to go to a chair to watch television and insisted she turn around and do the exercise. Is this abuse? Kate feels it is but is not sure what to do about it; she feels too intimidated to report it to anyone! What should she do?

3. Arthur loved his dogs and misses them very much. The manager of the home has decided that dogs cannot be allowed onto the premises for health and safety reasons. Arthur's daughter will no longer be able to bring them with her on her visits.

4. Jane's kosher meal has been discontinued because she doesn't seem bothered and often doesn't eat much of it. Because of her dementia she will eat practically anything when she is hungry.

5. Joe was always a very keen footballer and has always stayed up late on Saturdays to watch the football on television. However, the care staff on nights tell him the TV has to be off at 10.30pm.

6. Eric is not included on the day trip to the seaside because of his urinary incontinence and the possibility that he will have an accident.

Exercise 12.3

INSTITUTIONALISATION AS A FORM OF ABUSE

With a group of colleagues discuss whether or not you are doing things purely out of routine and in danger of becoming institutionalised yourselves. Are there areas of care where a more individualised approach could be adopted?

Chapter 13

Problem Solving and Trouble Shooting

Key messages

- The person with dementia is not being deliberately difficult.
- So-called 'problem behaviour' is realistic in the context of a dementia.
- Look for hidden meanings and underlying causes.
- There is always another way of doing something!

What is often called 'problem behaviour' can be more realistically interpreted as the efforts of the person with dementia to make sense of the strange and frightening world they find themselves in. Dementia renders the world a difficult place to live in. For them it must be a confusing world where less and less is recognisable or understandable. Memory loss, disorientation and failing cognitive abilities can result in clients feeling insecure and frightened, leading them to withdraw into a familiar and comforting past. Many will understandably rage against the bewildering world out of frustration and fear.

Trying to understand what it must be like to have dementia helps us to understand the behaviours it produces. Dementia can make people forget what is normal and what is not, what's acceptable in public and what's not, what's harmful and what's not. Stripping off in public may not be a problem for a client with dementia because they have forgotten social convention.

Sometimes difficult behaviours put the sufferer at risk, but often they do not – they are simply the result of our failure to adapt the environment or our practice to meet the client's psychological or other needs. There is always a reason and purpose behind 'problem behaviour'.

Bad practice avoids trying to understand the reasons behind behaviours and all too often results in over-reliance on tranquillising medication to 'solve' the problem. But it hasn't solved anything; it has merely eradicated the problem temporarily. Problem behaviours should not be 'managed' to get rid of them; rather they should be embraced as a challenge for us to try and find out what is wrong. Our goal should be to try to understand the person and their needs. How can we help to make life better so that the behaviour doesn't occur? We need to find the problem which is causing the problem behaviour and 'manage' that.

Discussion point

Imagine a complete stranger walks into your bedroom and mutters something you can't quite catch. They start to try to take off your clothes and to force you to get into a bath! Would you let them or would you do your best to resist and fight? An aggressive response would seem reasonable here!

The reaction of the client is often quite reasonable given the fact they have dementia. They are not being deliberately awkward.

Often behaviour which is apparently meaningless to us has real meaning for the client, especially if they are locked into a reality many years older than ours.

History

It is again clear that a good knowledge of the client and their history will forestall many problems. Knowing their likes and dislikes and routines will mean that your care can cater for their needs instead of ignoring them and causing problems.

Hidden meaning and underlying causes

There can be many possible and plausible explanations for 'problem behaviours'. The key to uncovering them is *observation*. You must assess the situation before you try and solve it and the only way to do this is to observe and watch what happens, listen to clients. The problem will present as a piece of one-off behaviour, you must monitor it over time and look for patterns and triggers (times of day, events, people). Think about *why* a behaviour is happening: why now, why this way, why this client? Exercise 13.3 (p.123) lists just a few explanations for you to consider. Some have simple solutions but others are not that obvious.

Back to basics

- Observe in order to assess.

- Look for the hidden meanings and possible underlying causes.

Trouble shooting

It is often useful to ask the following questions when faced with a problem:

- Is it really a problem – and why?

- Can it be broken down into sub-problems?

- What are the possible causes?

- Who is it a problem for? Client, family, other residents or just us (the answer to this will indicate quite different solutions)?

- Are we as carers unable or unwilling to adapt to it or accept it?

- Is it a problem because it just doesn't conform to our routine, expectations or values?

- Does the behaviour have a hidden meaning?

- Is the client trying to tell us something?

- What might be the underlying causes?

- Is the problem the problem, or is it the consequences?

- How can it be resolved in a way that brings least upset to the client?

It is useful to examine the problem on paper. Writing things down often helps to clarify the issues and focuses the mind.

Try drawing up two spider charts, one for 'causes' and another for 'consequences'.

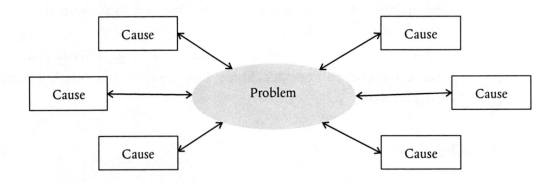

Figure 13.1 Exploring possible causes

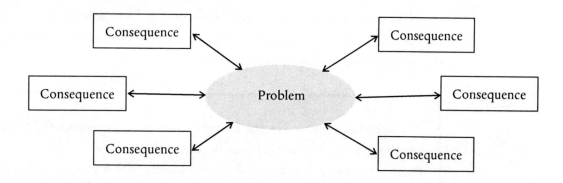

Figure 13.2 Exploring possible consequences

These will help you to explore further causes to tackle and also to look at whether it is the consequences that can be altered rather than the behaviour itself. When you have derived a list of possible causes, break this down even further and consider what factors might contribute to the cause (Figure 13.3). This will give you an even greater range of possible lines of solution.

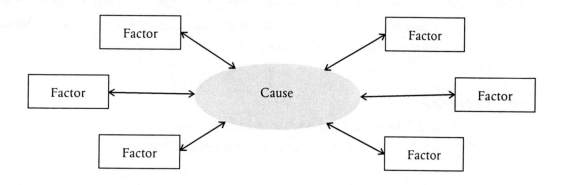

Figure 13.3 Exploring possible factors

Brain storm as many possibilities as you can to give you a wide range of explanations and solutions. It may not be the obvious issues which have to be addressed. Such an approach will also help you to adopt an individualised approach rather than just applying standard solutions.

Restating the problem

Sometimes you can be so involved with a problem it is hard to step back and see it objectively. This is why it is important to share it and seek the opinion of others. Get a group of colleagues together and spend some time explaining the problem you are having difficulty overcoming. Then ask the group to restate the problem in as many different ways as possible. This will help you to look at it from new directions and perspectives.

> Bill was a headmaster. He was keeping order, marking essays and praising staff and did not like not being shown his due respect. His wife felt he was happy on the ward because one day he had said to her, 'You know dear, this really is a rather good college'.

The person with dementia is never being deliberately difficult – slow and frustrating, maybe, but not deliberately difficult. They are just trying to cope in the best way they can. It is never their fault, they cannot be blamed for their illness. All too often it is we who are being deliberately fast, don't have the time and have lost the plot: that we are there to care. See the Trouble shooting summary on p.126 and Exercise 13.8 (p.127).

Health and Social Care National Occupational Standards

This chapter relates to many of the induction and foundation standards but in particular to the following level standards:

Level 2 core units

HSC21d Access and update records and reports.
HSC23 a + b Develop your knowledge and practice.

Level 2 optional units

HSC25 a, b + c Carry out and provide feedback on specific plan of care activities.
HSC224 a, b + c Observe, monitor and record the conditions of individuals.
HSC228 a, b + c Contribute to effective group care.
HSC241 a + b Contribute to the effectiveness of teams.

Level 3 core units

HSC33 a + b Reflect upon and develop your practice.

Level 3 optional units

HSC328 a, b + c Contribute to care planning and review.

Level 4 optional units

HSC416 a, b + c Develop, implement and review care plans with individuals.

Mental Health Standards

A1.1, 1.2 Develop your own knowledge and practice.

A2.1, 2.2 Reflect upon and develop practice using supervision and support.

A3.1, 3.2, 3.3 Promote the values and principles underpinning best practice.

Care Homes for Older People: National Minimum Standards

7.1 to 7.6 These standards relate to service users having a plan of care relating to their health, personal and social care needs and in which the service user is involved. Such plans should be reviewed monthly.

Further reading and references

Stokes, G. (2000) *Challenging Behaviours in Dementia: A Person Centred Approach.* Bicester: Speechmark. This whole book is excellent. It is full of insight and has useful case scenarios. See in particular Chapter 2 on assessment of behaviour in dementia and Chapter 7 'Taxonomies of possible explanations'.

✓

Exercise 13.1

TROUBLE SHOOTING

- Think about client behaviours in your workplace which cause the care staff problems.

- List each client's name on a flip chart and against it write down all those behaviours which are considered problematic or difficult.

- As a group, now try to come up with possible explanations for the behaviour. Think about the person's previous lifestyle, culture and work.

- What aspects of care might be frustrating to the client?

- What could you do about it?

Exercise 13.2

BILL: A CASE FOR CONSIDERATION

Bill used to pace around all the time. He was forever causing the nursing staff concern. He would stare at people fiercely, which they found intimidating, and he often refused to comply with requests centred around hygiene and eating. He couldn't be persuaded to do anything if he was 'that way out'. He would suddenly shout at other residents as they walked across his line of vision. Nurses muttered, 'It's as if he owns the place'. He would shout at people, pointing at them and giving them 'that look of disgust'. At other times he would sit quietly flicking through any old pile of papers or magazines and then come up to you and offer them to you and insist you took them. Resistance led him to get quite upset. On several occasions he would rearrange things, spending quite some time in getting it right, notices, ornaments, that sort of thing; he could be quite tidy. This used to get him into 'bother' as he would try to rearrange the television and fish tank, he needed watching! Every now and then though he would come up to you and, smiling, talk complete gibberish into your ear, look at you fondly and pat you on the back. Some of this was considered problem behaviour and some quite nice. It was all a mystery until, one day, a nurse thought to ask his wife what Bill used to do for a living.

Think about Bill's behaviours and what he does and try to guess what he might think he is doing. What occupation might make Bill's behaviours entirely understandable?

Exercise 13.3

CAUSES AND SOLUTIONS

For each possible cause discuss how you, as a team, can help the client to deal with it!

- Anger at their failing abilities.

- Being tired.

- Not being understood.

- Being depressed.

- Fear of what is happening to them.

- Needing the toilet, but not knowing where it is.

- Lack of privacy.

- Need for attention/companionship.

- Frustration.

- Not understanding what you want.

- Need for contact.

- Being ignored.

- Feelings not validated.

- Being cold.

- Boredom.

- Being too hot.

- Not being able to find their way around.

- People going too fast/being rushed.

- Missing their visitor.

- Malignant social psychology.

- A strange situation.

- Flashes of insight.

- Being prevented from doing what you want.

- Pain.

✓

- Discomfort.

- Not recognising things.

- Isolation.

- Feeling lost and unwanted, not belonging.

- Anxiety.

- Lost something.

- Not being sure where they are.

- Lack of choice.

- Physical problems such as constipation.

Exercise 13.4
BEHAVIOUR ROLE PLAY

One way of trying to get an understanding of what it is that is driving a piece of behaviour is to role play it.

- Choose any piece of behaviour which causes a problem for the care staff.

- Recreate the scenario with a colleague playing you and you role playing the client. Other staff should watch. This might sound silly and embarrassing, but it is an excellent method for inducing insight and therefore possible explanations and solutions.

- The staff member playing you can give feedback on how they felt the situation was handled and you can gain an insight into how it felt to be the client.

- This insight is twofold: you can get a feel for why the client might be behaving in this way and also what it feels like to be on the receiving end of care.

- Explore the feedback of those who watched and together generate some ideas to try.

Exercise 13.5

PROBLEM SCENARIO

'Come on, let's go!' Dave shouted back into the house. His wife Wendy looked on in horror from the hallway. There he was, standing outside in his pyjamas, halfway down the garden path, ready to go down to the supermarket for the weekly shop. He did not realise anything was wrong and felt he was appropriately dressed.

- What should Wendy do?

- What verbal response would help to diffuse the situation (brain storm as many as you can, they all have a chance of working – even, 'You silly man, have you seen yourself? A right sight you are!').

- What would lead to a confrontation and make matters much worse?

- How might you distract Dave?

Exercise 13.6

BEING REASONABLE!

In a group discuss:

- how often you need to take a bath

- how often you should change your shirt/blouse

- how often you should shave

- how often you should eat

- when the right times are for having cups of tea

- how often you should wash your hair and brush your teeth.

The point is, if clients do not want to do something, does it matter?

Exercise 13.7

TROUBLE SHOOTING SUMMARY

Here are some suggestions of what you can do when you feel a client's behaviour is problematic:

- Brain storm possible reasons and underlying causes.

- Look for hidden meanings, share and discuss them.

- Involve relatives and friends in finding a solution.

- Do not criticise or rebuke: the behaviour is not intended by the client to be difficult.

- There may be no answer – you cannot solve everything – but you can give comfort and reassurance and stay with the person, validating their experience.

- Do not expect the person to learn. You may have to go through the motions of your chosen solution every time.

- Just watch a behaviour and monitor it to gain a better understanding, rather than reacting to it immediately.

- Identify triggers and eradicate them.

- Do you need to refer to outside agencies or gain specialist advice?

- Is it cultural?

- Maintain a sense of humour.

- Offering reassurance and company might be the only thing you can do.

- What might be a workable compromise?

- Support your colleagues, take over from each other, relieve each other. Relax. Being fresh and relaxed aids tolerance and sometimes the behaviour just has to be tolerated.

- Try something new – relaxation and aromatherapy for example.

- Personalise – everyone is different and what worked for Joe will not necessarily work for Helen.

- Does it matter? Always a good question. Dementia demands the freedom to do things which seem very odd to the rest of us.

- Do nothing. Often the problem will go away.

Dementia Care Training Manual for Staff Working in Nursing and Residential Settings © Danny Walsh 2006

- Do nothing. Let it happen, but minimise the effects.

- Use distraction, such as suggesting a 'cup of tea' or a walk (but remember to validate real emotions and experiences and not just ignore them). It is a good crisis management strategy.

- Walk away. Often it is just a problem for you.

- Ask yourself, 'How would I like to be treated?'

Exercise 13.8

SCENARIO FOR DISCUSSION

Martin wanders restlessly for most of the day, but it's his pattern and he seems happy in this. However, he has grown into the habit of stripping off and wandering around half naked. This is upsetting some of the other residents. How would you go about resolving this?

Chapter 14

Wandering and Restlessness

Key message
Wandering is often meaningful, purposeful and not a problem to anyone.

Wandering and restlessness are common behaviours, which are often described as problematic, or as causing problems for care staff and other residents. However, when one examines the issues involved one can begin to see the 'problem' in a different light. In fact, often wandering is purposeful and not at all aimless, and in no way problematic if the reasons behind it are clearly understood (see Exercises 14.1 and 14.2, p.133).

Reasons

There can be many reasons why a client wanders and is restless and each reason points to a possible solution. Common reasons are:

- The confused person is lost.

- They need the toilet and cannot find it.

- They are experiencing pain or other physical discomfort, such as constipation.

- They are bored.

- They are enjoying the feeling of freedom wandering gives them.

- Medication sometimes can cause restlessness and agitation – check it.

- They may feel they are doing something, such as a job from their past.

- They might feel that it is time to go to work or pick the kids up!

- They may be lonely and in need of some attention and human contact.

- They are looking for a reassuring face.

- The person is bewildered and frightened by their lack of understanding of the world around them and their confusion. They might be trying to escape it.

- The person is seeking comfort: walking around a familiar route can be reassuring and so is purposeful.

- They may be anxious; anxiety can cause wandering and a restless pacing to and fro, a bit like rocking in a chair.

- They are looking for their visitor who has just left.

- They are hungry or thirsty.

- Often people can forget what it was they got up to do but continue wandering.

- It might be too noisy or busy for them.

- Habit.

- They are trying to get out because they can't understand why they are here.

- They are searching for things or people from the past.

Possible solutions to try

- Do nothing because most of the time there will be no need to intervene.

- Wander with the person if they appear upset, using touch and words as reassurance.

- Wander with the person if they are not upset in order to give company, acknowledge and boost feelings of worth.

- Everyone needs exercise, so plan daily walks and start an activity programme which is physically active. Wandering at night is often a result of lack of activity during the day.

- Do not make too many changes to a person's routine or environment. Remember that in dementia the familiar is reassuring. If a client has recently moved into a nursing home they may well be searching for familiar landmarks. Give them plenty of reassurance and contact and ensure that they have familiar personal possessions on view and try to maintain their personal routine.

- Create a safe wandering area such as an enclosed garden or a circular corridor route, where people can wander without hazard.

- Look at the person's history to see if there are reasons for wandering and clues to unmet needs.

- Darkness can be confusing and frightening. Much nocturnal wandering may be an attempt by the client to reassure themselves of where they are, so try subdued night lighting, so that they can easily see the areas they are likely to need during the night.

- Try Reality Orientation, such as using large signs and pictures to help orient the client to their surroundings and help them find rooms.

- Even when you cannot fathom the reason for the client's wandering and the person seems to be distressed, you should acknowledge and validate the feelings, explore them and reassure the client. Spending time with them will allow you the opportunity to pick up on clues whilst also giving comfort.

- Distraction is always a useful tool for defusing potentially difficult situations and simply suggesting a cup of tea will often work. However, it is important that in doing so we do not ignore the real feelings being expressed by the client. These can be explored and validated once the 'crisis' is over.

Medication and risk

Using sedative medication in an attempt to subdue restlessness is likely to make matters worse by increasing the risk of falls. Sedative medication is also sometimes used because the staffing levels are inadequate to ensure everyone's safety and so that carers can give each person the time they deserve. Used in this way medication is merely a form of restraint. It is far better to work out ways of allowing safe wandering. Often medication is used because we are worried about the patient's risk of falling. However, good care must carry with it an element of risk if we are not totally to sacrifice independence and freedom to safety. As always, discuss the issues as a team and consult family members in order to come up with a clear and agreed strategy.

Where wandering has led the client to become lost or wander out of the home it may still be possible to allow them to continue this freedom without undue risk. They can be provided with identity bracelets giving personal details and contact numbers. Try and establish a safe route for them to follow, such as to the local shop and back or just around the block. Inform local shopkeepers and neighbours that the client may become confused and give them your contact details. Always make a quick description of the clothing before they go for their walk, so that you have an accurate description if you need it. As always, it is a question of balancing safety and freedom and you will need to review the situation on a regular basis.

In cases where it is not possible to ensure safety and where the client continues to find their way outside and frequently becomes lost, other steps must be taken to ensure safety. Many homes have door entry systems such as key pads or baffle handles, so that clients cannot get out without asking a member of staff. Where systems like these are installed, care must be taken to ensure that the rights of other residents are not infringed and that this is done for safety reasons and not just out of convenience.

Health and Social Care National Occupational Standards

This chapter relates to many of the induction and foundation standards but in particular to the following level standards:

Level 2 core units

HSC21b Listen to and respond to individuals' questions and concerns.

HSC24b Treat people with respect and dignity.

HSC24c Assist in the protection of individuals.

Level 2 optional units

HSC216 a + b Help address the physical comfort needs of individuals.

HSC226 a, b + c Support individuals who are distressed.

HSC240 a, b + c Contribute to the identification of the risk of danger to individuals and others.

Level 3 core units

HSC32 a, b + c Promote, monitor and maintain health, safety and security in the working environment.

Level 3 optional units

HSC373 a, b + c Plan and implement programmes to enable individuals to find their way around unfamiliar environments.

HSC396 a, b + c Enable people with mental health needs to develop coping strategies.

Mental Health Standards

A4.1, 4.2 Promote effective communication and relationships.

A5.1, 5.2 Promote effective communication and relationships with people who are troubled or distressed.

J2.1, 2.2 Support individuals when they are distressed.

Care Homes for Older People: National Minimum Standards

10.5 Treat people with respect at all times.

14.1 This standard focuses on the service user's right to exercise autonomy and choice.

18.1 to 18.6 These standards are focused upon client protection. They aim to protect clients from physical, financial, psychological and sexual abuse, also from neglect and degrading treatment, whether through negligence or ignorance. The standards require safe procedures for responding to whistleblowers and the reporting of incidents of abuse.

Exercise 14.1

WANDERING: WHY IS IT A PROBLEM?

Harry worked as a fireman and is used to being up at all hours and being very active. He has worked out how to undo the baffle handles on the front doors of the nursing home. He tends to do it when it is just starting to get dark. He is usually found wandering around the block and has never become lost as yet.

- What might be the reasons for Harry's wandering?

- What would a good practice response be?

Exercise 14.2

WANDERING

- With a group of colleagues write a list of all the reasons you can think of as to why a person with dementia might be or appear to be wandering around aimlessly within *your* unit.

- There are, of course, many possible reasons and you should come up with a very lengthy list including some of the reasons given on pp.128–9.

- Now personalise the exercise by writing a list of those clients in your care who wander or are restless.

- Discuss why for some this is problematic and not for others.

- Who is it a problem for and why?

- Examine, for each client, what might be the reasons for their restlessness and discuss strategies for overcoming it if it is problematic.

Chapter 15

Accusations

Key messages
- Validate the feelings being expressed by the sufferer.
- Don't take it personally.

Alongside confusion and memory loss the fear and the frustration of failing mental powers that is felt by sufferers can lead to accusations implying that others are to blame for their losses and frightening feelings. There may be a frightening sense of being abandoned: 'Why aren't you helping me?' 'Why are you allowing this to go on?' 'Why are you doing this?'

It is important not to take such accusations personally and to try to reduce the obvious distress of the sufferer. Try to validate the emotions being displayed to give the client the comfort of knowing that you at least recognise that they are in such distress. If you can communicate such empathy then they will not feel so isolated.

Whilst accusations usually centre upon something being lost they can be more serious. Clients can believe that they are being burgled, that strangers are in 'their' house and that they are being abused (see Exercise 15.1, p.136).

Hiding and losing

Forgetting where things are is common and often leads to accusations of others moving or stealing things. We all know how frustrating it can be when, for example, we have not put our car keys down in the usual place. We can all identify with the rush of anxiety which occurs at the moment you realise that you can't find your wallet. These must be real and frequent sensations for our clients, often compounded by the conviction that someone has stolen them. It is a terrible state to be in.

Practical tips

- Help the person to look in the places things are normally kept as they may have lost this knowledge.

- Stay calm and don't argue as your own irritation will escalate the situation and increase their distress.

- Get to know the places clients put things as it can often be the same spot.

- Check the bins.

- Keep replacements of important things such as glasses, keys, etc.

- Hiding things may be an attempt by the client to stop change and loss and a realistic response to feelings of insecurity. Things are changing too quickly and they want to hang onto what they have left and so put things in a safe place. Clothes, for instance, may be hidden. The response needed here is one of reassurance and validation of the client's experience and feelings.

Health and Social Care National Occupational Standards

This chapter relates to many of the induction and foundation standards but in particular to the following level standards:

Level 2 core units

HSC21b Listen to and respond to individuals' questions and concerns.
HSC24b Treat people with respect and dignity.

Level 2 optional units

HSC226 a, b + c Supporting individuals who are distressed.

Level 3 core units

HSC31b Communicate effectively on difficult, complex and sensitive issues.

Mental Health Standards

A4.1, 4.2 Promote effective communication and relationships.
A6.1, 6.2, 6.3 Promote effective communication where there are communication differences.
A5.1, 5.2 Promote effective communication and relationships with people who are troubled or distressed.
J2.1, 2.2 Support individuals when they are distressed.

Care Homes for Older People: National Minimum Standards

10.5 Treating people with respect at all times.

✓

Exercise 15.1

MISUNDERSTANDINGS AND ACCUSATIONS

Imagine sitting at home one day relaxing in front of the television when two strangers grab you, march you to a cold white room and begin to strip you. They talk to each other in a foreign language. You resist, but they just smile at you and continue.

Handled badly this could easily become a nightmare scenario for the client.

- Identify the aspects of poor care involved here.

- How should the situation be managed from this point?

- What key skills are involved?

Dementia Care Training Manual for Staff Working in Nursing and Residential Settings © Danny Walsh 2006

Chapter 16

Aggression

Key messages

- Validate the feelings being expressed.
- Remember the person is confused.
- Most aggression is predictable and so avoidable.
- A good knowledge of your clients will allow much aggression to be avoided.

Aggression can be an extremely difficult problem to deal with. It is one which carers at home often struggle with yet, in nursing and residential homes, the problem is exacerbated by the presence of others whose interests must also be looked after.

Once again there are no clear-cut answers and guidelines that can be easily applied to magic the problem away. However, there are a number of ways of looking at aggression that can help us to understand its many causes. Doing so may help us to develop ways of eliminating those causes and of managing the aggression when it occurs.

Common causes of aggression

- Aggression rarely occurs without a reason, even in dementia. It is often a response to threatening circumstances or situations the sufferer does not understand.

- Aggression is not a continuous activity either, it occurs usually because of some trigger event. Carers should look for such triggers and chart what, where and when aggression occurs. They should consider what was happening to the person immediately prior to the aggression. In doing this, carers can move closer to the answer to the question: why?

- Common reasons for aggression in dementia are the sufferers lack of understanding about what is going on around them. The fear, frustration and feelings of anxiety this must bring about are reason enough to form an aggressive response when staff try to 'do things for the person'. However, it must be very hard for relatives to come to terms with such aggression, and they can feel rejected despite all they have done for the person – especially if that person was previously quite passive.

Other common causes are:

- Fear at no longer recognising places, people or purpose, such as forgetting why you are doing something.

- Frustration at dependency upon others and at failure at simple tasks.

- Where the client has insight, the impact of their losses can be devastating and resistance to being 'helped' is a logical response.

- Being unable to express what you want or no one understanding what you say.

- Humiliation at loss of dignity and having to have things done for you.

- Lack of dignity or respect for it.

- Feeling patronised.

- Losing the ability to control feelings and anger (dementia can remove this ability), so that increasing frustration erupts into aggression.

- Insight, fear at loss of power and control in life; realisation of loss of failing mental powers.

- Lack of attention, feeling rejected.

- Inability to make sense of and misunderstanding what's going on.

- Being frightened.

- Inappropriate care (malignant social psychology).

- Having your personal space invaded by an apparent stranger and not understanding why. In this context, as in many of the others, the aggression is a realistic response.

- Being asked questions you can't answer. Assessments often result in irritability, if not aggression, as the client's frustration boils over.

- Where insight is present clients may be afraid of being exposed to others realising they have failing cognitive powers and a poor memory. Hence they are angry at assessments and make accusations about others in an attempt to lay the blame elsewhere.

- Being tired.

- Design and routine of the nursing home. What is there about the design and routine of your home that might contribute to aggressive outbursts?

Most of the causes cited for wandering can also be included, such as pain and discomfort, etc.

Interventions and ideas

- *Stay calm* – Agitation on your part will be picked up by the client through your non-verbal signals, which will signal to the client a lack of reassurance and a degree of uncertainty. This will help to prolong and exacerbate the aggression. Don't raise your voice.

- *Do nothing* – Walk away and count to 100. Often aggression resolves itself and intervening only serves to make an issue of it.

- *Don't argue* – This will only pour oil on the flames. Count to 10, then 30. Convey warmth and reassurance via the tone of your voice. Above all, do not interpret the aggression as if it comes from someone without dementia. It is not personal: the client is frightened or feeling vulnerable or angry and you just happen to be there. Regard it as an opportunity to do some good by soaking it up and changing the feelings of fear into ones of security.

- *Don't touch* – This can easily be misinterpreted as aggression on your part. Don't attempt to lead the person away as this can also be misinterpreted as assault; doing so additionally gives the message that you have not listened or don't care about why the person is angry.

- *Facilitate verbal aggression* – Allow the client to express their anger verbally and to get their feelings out of their system. Often this is all that is required. Listen and validate the anger because to stifle it at this stage is likely to escalate it into possible physical aggression. When you ignore an angry person, they become more incensed.

- *Give space* – Do not crowd an aggressive person: keep a distance and do not invade their body space.

- *Others* – Direct others away from the scene or direct the person away from others. Aggression is easier to deal with in the absence of an audience and an audience can make it harder for an aggressor to back down.

- *Prevention* – Prevention begins by reducing the demands upon the sufferer when they are showing signs of stress. Similarly, creating an unpressured culture in an unrushed, stress-free environment will help. Allow time for clients to succeed and slow down in communication to give them time to think about what has been said and to formulate a response. Create opportunities for success.

- *Seek hidden meanings and underlying causes* – Always look for the triggers and causal events, the reasons for the aggression. Attempts to understand causes will always foster new insights and thus ways of dealing with the situation. Try to unearth the hidden meanings behind behaviour, remembering that there is seldom no reason.

- *Validate the anger* – Show that you recognise the client's anger, as to ignore it is to devalue their feelings and can make matters worse if the client feels their concerns are being ignored.

- *Validate the meaning* – You also need to listen to and engage the client in whatever is the reality for them. So validate the content of what they are saying by relating to it and discussing it.

- *Talk* – Reassure people that you want to help them and will stay with them to sort 'it' out. Speak gently and ask them what the matter is – this shows you are concerned. Say you want to help.

- *Key worker* – If possible try to get a key worker or someone the client knows well or has a good relationship with to talk to them. A familiar, reassuring face can often de-escalate the situation.

- *Distraction* – A last resort but a useful tool. You should always try to validate the client's feelings first and seek to address underlying causes. However, when all else fails, it may be useful to try distraction. Suggesting having a drink or suggesting a different activity can help to take the focus away from the aggression. Propose activities the client enjoys. The poor short-term memory of dementia plays a part here and episodes are often quickly forgotten. Sometimes a fresh friendly face taking over the situation is enough to distract and calm things down.

Remember:

- It is not the person but the disease.

- It is not personal.

- Tone of voice and non-verbals are crucial.

- Look for the cause.

- We are all novices – the clients are the experts.

- Ensure all strategies are written up in the care plans.

Health and Social Care National Occupational Standards

This chapter relates to many of the induction and foundation standards but in particular to the following level standards:

Level 2 core units

HSC21b Listen to and respond to individuals' questions and concerns.

HSC24b Treat people with respect and dignity.

HSC24c Assist in the protection of individuals.

Level 2 optional units

HSC226 a, b + c Support individuals who are distressed.

HSC232 a + b Protect yourself from the risk of violence at work.

HSC240 a, b + c Contribute to the identification of the risk of danger to individuals and others.

Level 3 core units

HSC31b Communicate effectively on difficult, complex and sensitive issues.

HSC32 a, b + c Promote, monitor and maintain health, safety and security in the working environment.

Level 3 optional units

HSC336 a, b + c Contribute to the prevention and management of abusive and aggressive behaviour.

HSC395 a, b + c Contribute to assessing and act upon risk of danger, harm and abuse.

HSC396 a, b + c Enable people with mental health needs to develop coping strategies.

Mental Health Standards

A4.1, 4.2 Promote effective communication and relationships.

A6.1, 6.2, 6.3 Promote effective communication where there are communication differences.

A5.1, 5.2 Promote effective communication and relationships with people who are troubled or distressed.

J2.1, 2.2 Support individuals when they are distressed.

Care Homes for Older People: National Minimum Standards

10.5 Treat people with respect at all times.

18.1 to 18.6 These standards are focused upon client protection. They aim to protect clients from physical, financial, psychological and sexual abuse. Also from neglect and degrading treatment, whether through negligence or ignorance. The standards require safe procedures for responding to whistleblowers and the reporting of incidents of abuse.

Exercise 16.1

AGGRESSION

- Think about the person with dementia and what it must be like to be that person.

- With your colleagues try to come up with as many reasons as you can why that person might become aggressive.

- Write them down on a flip chart.

- Next, again with your colleagues, write a list of all your clients who are classed as aggressive.

- Think about each client and come up with reasons as to why they have this label.

- Think about aspects of the home, the routine and the care, which might contribute to this.

Having got this far, it is pertinent to use the exercise to seek some solutions. As a group, brain storm ways in which you might do or arrange things differently to increase the client's level of comfort and reduce the level of aggression.

✓

Exercise 16.2

OUR OWN INSIGHT AND SKILLS

In a group of colleagues, write a list of things that make you angry. Include the big things such as world poverty and wars, but also write down the little things which might appear trivial to others but are important to you – people not being on time or untidiness. Be honest and generate a full list.

When finished contemplate just how big and varied the list is. Think about how long it might take you to unearth this range of responses as possible reasons for aggression from clients and how long it might take to get to the bottom of why a client is angry. Next consider how you react when you are angry and what actions by others help you to regain a state of calm!

This is the beginnings of a list of strategies which can be added to by asking the group how they defuse awkward situations and to give examples of aggressive situations they have been involved with. Discuss what might and might not work with clients with a dementia.

Exercise 16.3

AGGRESSION SCENARIOS TO CONSIDER

1.   Jennifer was admitted to the nursing home three weeks ago. She is confused and doesn't know why she is there. She is upset and feels she has been kidnapped. She insists she has to go and 'pick the kids up' and tries to get out of the front door. A care assistant tries to stop her, saying, 'It's all right Jennifer, come and have a cup of tea'. Jennifer becomes verbally aggressive and upset and, as the care assistant tries to steer her away, Jennifer hits out.

   • What are the underlying feelings for Jennifer?

   • How might the situation have been handled differently?

2.   Peter was a big chap and physically quite intimidating. A Yorkshireman through and through, he had worked on the land and lived by simple rules. He did not suffer fools gladly and often shouted at those he thought were a nuisance. Peter was especially frustrated at his loss of communication. His key worker had got to know him very well, so much so that, whenever Peter became aggressive as his abilities declined and his insight remained, the key worker would just go up to him and put his arms around him and give him a hug.

   • Why is this good practice?

   • What effects does it have?

3.   Dave had just hit another resident but, rather than isolate him and tell him off, his key worker reassured him and asked him if he was all right and what was bothering him.

   • Why is this good practice?

4.   Mrs Gray enjoys the free time she gets when her husband attends the day centre at the local nursing home. One day she turns up with a bruise to her cheek. 'He hit me', she tells the nurse. 'I was only trying to get him dressed and he was being awkward, and I told him so.'

   • What advice would you give to Mrs Gray?

Chapter 17

Disinhibition

Key messages
- Disinhibition is often a plea for affection and company.
- People with dementia still have sexual needs and rights.

A large number of people with dementia may lose interest in sexual activity. However, for many others, sexual desires persist well into the advanced stages.

Convention

The recognition of convention and norms can be lost in dementia. Undressing in public is not recognised as taboo. Such behaviours can be dealt with by simply redirecting the client to a private area. As cognitive decline proceeds, some factors which usually inhibit our sexual behaviour can be eroded and the expression of sexual desires can become unacceptably overt.

Physical affection

There is often a lack of physical contact and physical affection in care home settings and many clients can miss this intimacy. Everybody is different but, if you have been tactile all your life and now find yourself alone in the world, or seemingly so, it is natural to try to regain some intimate contact. We need to identify those with these needs and ensure they receive regular doses of hugs, kisses, hand-holding, sitting with, cuddles etc.

Sex

An expression of sexual desire is hardly ever seen as a positive thing in our client group. This fact alone highlights our reluctance to embrace the reality. Sex is an important part of most of our lives and a desire which can remain long into a dementia. It is normal for older people to need sex. Often the problem arises from our inability to accept this and to call this need problematic behaviour. The lack of sex becomes an unmet need and, because it is a basic biological urge, its unfulfillment can lead to frustration. The loss of recognition of social and sexual conventions can lead to awkward situations, but the person is only doing what feels good and natural. Sexual desire where it continues should be allowed to be fulfilled in privacy if at all possible.

Difficulties can also arise out of our giving misleading impressions, stemming from an assumption that older people are not sexually interested. If you were a woman wearing a low-cut blouse, would you lean over a 20-year-old male client in the same way you would with a 70-year-old gentleman? If you assume that sexual needs are lost it is easy to fall into the trap of thinking that your close affection will not be wrongly interpreted. So we need to provide affection and warmth but we need to be careful about what signals we give off. Remember too that many clients with dementia are locked into the past and may regard themselves as much younger than they are – and behave accordingly. The dress code of today is very much more provocative than it was 50 years ago.

Expressing sexuality

Expressing sexuality can remain a prime need. It is important to be allowed to be what you are, and so opportunity should be made for clients to express and reaffirm their sexuality. Dances and special occasions are good opportunities for this. Putting on smart clothes and getting dressed up, wearing make-up and having your hair done will all help this goal. Dances allow for further reaffirmation of masculinity or femininity and provide the opportunity for clients to be chivalrous, rakish, coy, flirty, etc. in keeping with their personalities.

Rudeness and swearing

Commonly rudeness arises out of frustration. The frustration needs to be acknowledged and validated and the cause needs to be identified. If you tell the person off you will miss the opportunity to explore and validate their feelings; you may also make matters worse. In public such behaviour can be embarrassing and it may be that you have to explain to other people and other clients that the person is ill and that the remark was not intended as a personal affront.

Family

Where problems are perceived the family should be invited to participate in care planning and case conferences. The family who visit may well be able to help in providing some form of intimate personal care. Help them by suggesting ways in which they could become involved, such as bathing, hair care, beauty treatment, massage, etc. This personal giving of intimate care might well fill the need for physical contact and indeed sexual contact, which if left can surface as frustration.

Validation

Mabel is 77 and very much a flirt. She constantly tells carers that she has been 'walking out' with some of the male residents and talks about dating. Most carers dismiss her and tell her not to tell lies, at which point she usually burst into tears. One carer though takes the time to ask her about her dates and they sit swapping stories and discussing old flames. In doing so she validates Mabel's world and makes her feel real.

Tactics

- Remember it is the dementia not the person.

- Remember that sexual needs are normal in older people. Do not fall into the trap of being ageist.

- Be aware of the need to comfort and protect other clients. Are they intimidated or distressed in any way?

- Use distraction if appropriate.

- Engage clients in meaningful activity, regularly and frequently.

- Ask the question, 'Is this behaviour sexual?', or is there some other driving force or reason?

- Involve the family.

- Make provision for fulfillment of sexual needs in privacy.

- Provide physical affection via kisses, hand-holding, sitting with, cuddles, closeness, hand massage, etc.

- Don't rebuke the client, calmly explain the situation.

- Protect the dignity of the disinhibited.

- Stripping in public is often indicative of discomfort due to ill-fitting clothes or a need for the toilet.

- Genital fondling may be indicative of the need for affection and physical contact or companionship.

- Ask, 'Who is the behaviour a problem for?' This will determine the nature of your response.

Health and Social Care National Occupational Standards

This chapter relates to many of the induction and foundation standards but in particular to the following level standards:

Level 2 core units

> HSC24 a, b + c Ensure your own actions support the care, protection and well being of individuals.

Level 3 optional units

> HSC397 a + b Reinforce positive behavioural goals during relationships with individuals.
>
> HSC398 a, b + c Contribute to assessing the needs of individuals for therapeutic programmes to enable them to manage their behaviour.

Mental Health Standards

> A4.1, 4.2 Promote effective communication and relationships.
>
> A5.1, 5.2 Promote effective communication and relationships with people who are troubled or distressed.
>
> J2.1, 2.2 Support individuals when they are distressed.

Care Homes for Older People: National Minimum Standards

> 10.1, 10.5, 10.7 These relate to privacy needs of clients.

✓

Exercise 17.1

SCENARIOS TO CONSIDER IN GROUPS

- Lenny is a fairly new resident at the home and he is not settling in very well. He tends to isolate himself and will not join in any activity. Often he is to be found sitting in an armchair in a quiet corner with his hands down his trousers fondling his genitals.

- Shirley is forever removing her dress and walking into the lounge as if nothing is wrong.

- Harry regularly sits in an armchair in the middle of the lounge and takes out his penis and begins to masturbate. He shouts at the women and leers across the room. A visitor complains about Harry and says that Harry is upsetting their mother. How would you deal with this and what would you say to them?

- Julie often sits next to care workers and begins to caress their arms and hold their hands. She does this with other residents too. She just sits there caressing them and smiling.

For each scenario brain storm a likely list of reasons for the behaviour. Write them down on a flip chart and for each reason come up with an action plan to resolve the situation.

Exercise 17.2
ETHICAL DILEMMAS

Often what is morally correct can be against the law and likewise what is legal can be morally wrong. Ethics does not give us answers to tricky problems but does give us different ways of looking at them. Discuss the following hypothetical scenarios in a group and try to come up with acceptable solutions which are also happy outcomes!

- Jenny regularly pesters male residents for sexually oriented affection. The male residents do not respond or understand and her daughter is totally distraught that her mother could act in this way. She feels that such behaviour is an insult to her late father.

- Danny forms a relationship with Susan, both of whom live in your nursing home. Neither has dementia, they are just a bit frail. Both are sexually active and they have begun to disappear into each other's rooms frequently. One day a member of staff walks in on them having intercourse. There is embarrassment all round. Think about your responses if it was the same scenario but both had moderate dementia.

- Mark asks to be taken to the newsagent. He wants to buy some pornographic magazines to help him meet his sexual needs. Should we help him to access videos?

- Arthur rings a local 'escort service' to hire a girl who arrives at the home and duly takes Arthur into his room. This is hypothetical of course, but if prostitution was legal, should the client not have the right to spend his money how he chooses?

Chapter 18

Dressing

Key messages

- Most problems with dressing occur because we try to rush clients.
- Appearance is not that important!

Difficulties with dressing can be especially frustrating for carers because they occur at times when there is often much else to do. People with dementia often find dressing quite taxing because there are so many steps involved. It is easy for us to take it for granted, but the simple task of putting your shoes on can be broken down into many separate tasks, some of which are quite tricky, such as fastening your laces. People with dementia can forget how to dress, what order garmets should go on or how many layers they should wear. They can get things on back to front and get frustrated with clips and buttons they can't manage. Often they can't appreciate the need for specific types of clothing, such as warm clothes on cold days. They also might not recognise the need to change their clothes when dirty or at bedtime.

Trouble shooting

- Does it matter? If a client insists on wearing two pairs of trousers during the day or an overcoat to sleep in, if it is doing them no harm, why intervene? Whose problem is it?

- Break the task down and lay out or present clothes in the order they are to be put on.

- Present only a limited number of choices, for example, do you want to wear the red one or the blue one today?

- Keep instructions short and focused on one thing at a time, such as 'Put your leg through here'.

- Mime the actions as this will provide clues and act as a trigger.

- Talk to the client the whole time.

- Make sure there are no distractions.

- Take dirty clothes away at every opportunity so the chance to put them back on is reduced.

- Try to keep to the client's previous routine and habits. If they always got dressed after washing, or put their clothes on in a certain order, then adhere to this pattern.

- Pay attention to comfort and privacy, ensuring that there will be no disturbances and that the room is warm. People with dementia are often reluctant to get undressed in front of another person they do not know.

- Choose clothes which will not need ironing and be aware of practicalities such as the use of slip-on shoes.

- If a person always wants to wear the same thing, get several copies of it.

- There may be some physical illness which is manifesting itself in the inability to get dressed or in lethargy. Consult the client's GP.

- Ensure that the client's vision is good.

- Check for depression. This is common in the early stages of dementia when some insight gives the sufferer a disturbing glimpse of their failing powers. In depression the sufferer loses interest in their personal hygiene and the need to look presentable. We need to be alert to the signs of depression. If you feel that a client may be depressed then you should contact the GP or community psychiatric nurse.

Independence

Assistance should focus on maintaining independence and giving choice. Try to allow clients to choose the clothes they wear; perhaps you might have to lay a selection out for them and help them to choose, but at least you are involving them in the process. You also might need to adapt clothes and make use of such aids as Velcro so that clients can more easily undo them and get them on and off. Lay the clothes out in the order that they should be put on or hand them to the person one at a time and guide them through the process. Try using prompts and mime.

Make dressing time an enjoyable interaction rather than a chore to be got through. To do this you will have to make time so as not to rush the client through the process, and possibly end up doing it yourself, de-skilling them in the process and subjecting them to feelings of failure. The whole dressing process is an opportunity to boost confidence and make people feel good about themselves. It is an opportunity to interact positively and give praise.

Details

Remember the little extras which go a long way to making a difference.

- After getting the client dressed help them to do their hair.

- Find out what preferences they had for hairsprays and other products or ornaments.

- Did they like to apply perfumes or deodorants?

- What sort of other details were important to them?

- Did they wear jewellery?

- When and how did they like to shave?

- When did they do their nails?

- Did they visit the toilet before or after dressing or breakfast?

- Did they do nothing until they had a cup of tea?

These are small details but ones which, if accounted for, will make a huge difference to the client's feelings of well-being and contentment.

Health and Social Care National Occupational Standards

This chapter relates to many of the induction and foundation standards but in particular to the following level standards:

Level 2 optional units

HSC29b Support individuals to identify and obtain household and personal goods.
HSC218c Support individuals in personal grooming and dressing.

Level 3 core units

HSC35b Respect the diversity and difference of individuals.

Level 4 optional units

HSC414a Work with individuals to assess their needs and preferences.

Care Homes for Older People: National Minimum Standards

10.3 Service users to wear their own clothes at all times.
10.5, 10.7 These relate to privacy needs of clients.
14.1 The home maximises the service user's capacity to exercise personal autonomy and choice.

DIFFICULTY WITH DRESSING

Terry doesn't mean to be difficult but he just can't grasp what is meant to be going on. He is getting a reputation for being 'difficult', especially in the morning. When you try to help him to get dressed he obliges you while you are directly next to him, and he lets you help him put clothes on. However, as soon as you turn around he starts taking them off again. Staff find this very frustrating and are apt to be rather brusque with him in order to get the job done. This clearly upsets Terry, who then becomes aggressive.

From another point of view, you wake up, in a strange room and a woman you do not recognise comes into the room. You don't know who she is or where you are. She touches you, pulling at you, she tries to force you into a bag. You take it off and she puts it back over your head. Next she forces something onto your feet and is talking gibberish.

- Why do care workers find situations like Terry's particularly difficult?

- What tactics and approaches might the care workers use in this scenario?

Chapter 19

Eating and Nutrition

Key messages

- It is important to know your client's history.
- Giving time will overcome many problems.
- Let the client do as much for themselves as possible.
- There are lots of different ways to eat. You don't necessarily have to sit down to a meal and it doesn't really matter when you eat.

Recognising the need to eat and the social conventions surrounding food can all be eroded by dementia. Many will forget to eat or that they have just eaten and it may be as difficult to get some to stop eating as it is to encourage others to eat well. Sufferers can develop some bizarre diets and strange eating timetables and habits, but if they are remaining well and not suffering so be it. In institutional settings you will often need to strike a balance between allowing odd eating habits due to disinhibition and declining coordination, and protecting the dignity of fellow residents. You do not want to strip a resident of their independence but you might have to arrange a separate eating schedule or area in order to satisfy all concerned. Remember, the undignified eater is at risk of being an outcast so you have a duty to protect them from this social disapproval.

Fluids

You can survive for quite a few weeks without food, but without water you would not last very long at all. With a reduced fluid intake you will suffer all sorts of physical complications. Dehydration is also a major cause of confusion and a reduced fluid intake greatly increases the chances of a urinary tract infection. We are supposed to take in about 1500ml of water a day. That is the equivalent of ten cups of water a day. A drink with every meal and one between would not achieve this so we need to be proactive in ensuring fluid levels are maintained. Often care assistants will be called upon to help clients to drink. The use of spouted cups and child feeders is common and is a realistic way of overcoming the problems.

Possible solutions

- Be certain that the person cannot do things for themselves.

- Eating with the clients is often frowned upon or not allowed in institutional settings and yet if you do it will encourage the clients. You may be acting as a role model as well as providing an opportunity for some social interaction. This is particularly helpful for those clients who have forgotten what to do with the food: they may not recognise it as such, but they might follow your example.

- It does not matter if a hot meal is not taken every day, cold foods such as sandwiches are equally nutritious.

- Often the client will wander away from the table and simply redirecting them back to the table is enough to jog their memories that they are eating!

- Just sitting with the client and helping them with food can be enough.

- When the client has lost the ability to use cutlery or will not stay at the table, try providing finger foods such as sausage rolls and bars which can be handled and eaten on the move.

- The provision of finger foods also helps to preserve some independence.

- If clients do not mind you feeding them, then this is a useful option. But ensure you are not doing this for the sake of saving time.

- When feeding a client never stand over them, sit down besides them and talk to them. Check to ensure that food has been swallowed. Talk to the person and ask what they want next: 'Do you want some sausage next?'

- Ensure that the pace of feeding is right.

- Where chewing and swallowing difficulties arise. Allow clients to take their time; it does not necessarily matter if the food gets cold.

- You may have to consider a soft or liquidised diet in order to preserve a client's independence, but still have due regard for presentation.

- Where food is refused, encourage snacks and drink supplements.

- Sometimes you might just need to place food into the client's mouth to start them off. There are many halfway houses between independent feeding and being fed.

- Ensure plenty of activity during the day, to work up an appetite.

- Get an occupational therapist to assess the client for the possibility of feeding aids, such as easy-to-hold cutlery and high-sided plates: these can greatly prolong independence.

- The timing of the meal may be wrong for the client.

- Clients may not like the food.

- Food may be too hot or too cold, too runny or too thick!

- The client may be preoccupied with other concerns. Do not force people to eat but return later and try again.

- Beware of constipation and ensure enough roughage and exercise are taken.

- For those whose declining nutrition is becoming problematic, enlist the help of a dietician who can advise on the best foods to offer and what drink supplements to give.

- Notions of a healthy diet might have to be ignored in dementia where clients are struggling to retain weight. The emphasis here might be on getting them to eat high-calorie foods, especially if they are eating very little at all.

- Know your client so that you are aware of favourite foods to offer them. Food tastes are acquired over a long period of time, a lifetime in fact, so they are not easily going to be changed. Ask relatives.

- The habit of eating in a large room with many other people is not easy to get used to.

- Try to ensure that there are no distractions at mealtimes.

- Be aware of cultural or religious needs in relation to food.

- Check that dentures fit and teeth are cared for.

Fun

Mealtimes should be fun and occasions for socialisation. In summer do not miss the opportunity to eat al fresco and create a party atmosphere. Make the dining room cheerful, like a restaurant, with table cloths, candles, flowers etc. Engage clients in tasks relating to mealtimes, such as setting the tables and helping to prepare food. Occasionally have themed nights or parties which the clients can help prepare for.

> **Discussion point**
>
> Mealtimes can be the best part of the day for many clients and something they look forward to or always enjoy. It is worth spending some time and energy to keep this state of affairs going.
>
> Think about the mealtime routine in your institution and come up with ways of de-institutionalising it. How can you make it less formal and more personal?

Health and Social Care National Occupational Standards

This chapter relates to many of the induction and foundation standards but in particular to the following level standards:

Level 2 optional units

HSC213 a, b + c Provide food and drink for individuals.
HSC214 a, b + c Help individuals to eat and drink.

Level 3 core units

HSC35b Respect the diversity and difference of individuals.

Level 4 optional units

HSC414a Work with individuals to assess their needs and preferences.

Care Homes for Older People: National Minimum Standards

12.1 and 12.2 These relate to choice and flexibility in relation to mealtimes and food.

14.1 The home maximises the service user's capacity to exercise personal autonomy and choice.

15.1 to 15.9 All relate to meals and mealtimes and focus on the outcomes of ensuring a balanced diet in a congenial setting, at times suited to the client.

✓

Exercise 19.1
EATING DIFFICULTY SCENARIOS

- Pamela is causing the staff some concern. She obviously enjoys her food but frequently chews it for several minutes and then takes it out of her mouth and places it neatly on the table.

- Keith never seems to need to eat; he is always reluctant and has to be almost forced to the table and fed. Frequently he will sit still and spit out anything you try to give him. You are concerned that he is not getting enough nourishment and that the other residents are not being allowed the right of a dignified mealtime.

These are just two examples of many feeding and nutrition dilemmas which can occur in dementia. As a group, work your way through the trouble shooting process to come up with possible reasons and solutions.

Exercise 19.2
YOUR CLIENTS

Make a list of your own clients and for each one list any eating problems they might have, then any nutritional deficits; identify what their favourite foods are and also what drinks they like. Next identify what they like as a special treat. Having done this for each client, write a section for each client's care plan outlining feeding preferences and nutritional guidelines.

Chapter 20

Hallucinations

Key messages
- Check for sensory deficits such as hearing difficulties.
- Validate feelings and comfort the sufferer.

Some clients with dementia may have hallucinations, but there may also be other explanations for what appears to be a hallucination. The commonest hallucinations are auditory and visual, but they can affect the other senses of smell, taste and touch. Hallucinations can be disturbing and frightening and clients will need a good deal of comforting and reassurance.

Trouble shooting

- Clarify that it is a hallucination and not just a misinterpretation of another stimulus, such as strange shadows on the curtains at night, or leaves tapping at the windows. Make sure that there is adequate lighting to reduce the risk of misinterpretation.

- Check for sensory deficits with ear and eye tests.

- Do not collude with a hallucination by suggesting that you too can hear or see it.

- Do not dismiss it by telling the client that there is really nothing there. To do this is to invalidate their reality and hallucinations are very real to experience. When others deny their existence it can make the sufferer feel very alone and afraid.

- Validate the feelings. Whilst we cannot see or hear hallucinations we can appreciate how disturbing they must be. So it is important to offer comfort and reassurance.

- Being with the person and holding their hand or putting your arms around them will be very comforting and give the message you are concerned. Remain with the person until the distress has gone. Affection alleviates distress.

- Tell the client you will stay with them and make sure no harm comes to them. A calm tone of voice helps.

- If the client cannot be reassured then it might be possible to distract them onto an activity which will break off the link with the hallucination.

- Activity is a good preventative for hallucinations. Inactivity allows a hallucination to take the sufferer's full attention. They will have less impact if people are busy.

- Where hallucinations persist it is worth getting medical advice regarding the use of anti-psychotic medicines. These can be effective in moderate doses but tranquillising at higher ones. It is also worth checking for other medical causes such as infections, dehydration and the side effects of other drugs.

Health and Social Care National Occupational Standards

This chapter relates to many of the induction and foundation standards but in particular to the following level standards:

Level 2 core units

HSC24 a, b +c Ensure your actions support the care, protection and well being of individuals.

Level 2 optional units

HSC226 a, b + c Support individuals who are distressed.

Mental Health Standards

A5.1, 5.2 Promote effective communication and relationships with people who are troubled or distressed.

Chapter 21

Toileting Difficulties and Incontinence

Key messages
- Recognise clients' individual needs and body language.
- Use the trouble shooting process.

There are many possible causes of toileting difficulties and incontinence and the key to overcoming the problem is, once again, knowing your client. Sometimes clients simply forget where the toilet is or forget to go to the toilet. Sometimes it is simply because they cannot undo their clothing or can't find the toilet at night. Many clients will have their own signs and behaviours which will alert you to the fact that they need the toilet.

Clients who are incontinent and who retain a degree of insight will often feel ashamed and are in urgent need of reassurance. The shame which must be felt at this stage can lead to clients trying to conceal their accidents. They are trying to cope with their problems as best they can. They can panic, not knowing where to dispose of their accidents. This is especially upsetting for them if they have soiled and they can sometimes try to hide the evidence by putting it in places they think it will not be found. For carers this can be especially difficult, but we must always try to focus on the feelings and fears of the client who has been moved to the desperate measure of hiding their accidents.

Trouble shooting

- Observe and record when people need the toilet and plot toileting routines according to this pattern rather than having mass toileting sessions at times not suited to many individuals.

- Use gentle reminders.

- Ensure appropriate night-time lighting and access to the toilet. Check that they can get out of the bed and that it is not too high.

- Try placing a commode in the bedroom.

- Offer the opportunity to visit the toilet regularly and especially last thing at night.

- Learn to recognise clients' behaviours. When the need for toileting arises clients will often display distinct behaviour patterns, such as restlessness, fidgeting or pulling at clothes, indicating anxiety.

- When a client appears to be wandering aimlessly try taking them to the toilet, as it may be that they are looking for it.

- Clients may mistake other objects for the toilet such as the sink or bin. Be alert to this and redirect as necessary.

- Is there a need for Reality Orientation to preserve independence? Has the client just lost the recognition of the toilet or where it is and do you need to provide a sign or picture on the door?

- Try fastenings such as Velcro or elasticated waistbands so that clients can easily undo their clothing and thus remain independent.

- Is incontinence due to lack of privacy?

- Use pads and other aids only to preserve dignity and independence and to allow undisturbed sleep. Ensure that they are changed regularly and that a care plan is invoked to maintain good skin care. Ask the incontinence advisor about the latest good skin care methods.

- Reduce late night liquid intake.

- Check for infections such as urinary tract infections and other medical conditions, such as constipation, which might be responsible. Urinary tract infections usually turn the urine dark and render it quite pungent.

- Ensure that incontinence is not due to medication such as diuretics used for high blood pressure, or sedatives.

- Chart incontinence; this will highlight any patterns emerging and individual needs. In institutions toileting can often occur 'en masse' at prescribed times and this ignores individual routines and preferences.

- Contact the continence advisory nurse or incontinence specialist of the local NHS trust to gain advice regarding help, products and useful interventions or techniques.

Health and Social Care National Occupational Standards

This chapter relates to many of the induction and foundation standards but in particular to the following level standards:

Level 2 optional units

> HSC218a Support individuals to go to the toilet.
>
> HSC219 a + b Support individuals to manage continence.

Level 3 optional units

> HSC372 a, b + c Plan and implement programmes for individuals to find their way around familiar environments.
>
> HSC373 a, b + c Plan and implement programmes for individuals to find their way around unfamiliar environments.

Care Homes for Older People: National Minimum Standards

> 10.1, 10.5, 10.7 These relate to privacy needs of clients.
>
> 21.1 to 21.9 These relate to lavatories and washing facilities and require that they are accessible, clearly marked and en suite.

✓

Exercise 21.1

INCONTINENCE PROBLEM

Simon is a joy to be with, quiet in nature and always smiling. He is only mildly demented and appears happy. He is, however, frequently incontinent of urine. A nurse suggests that you try pads but he pulls them out as soon as you have put them on him and he is going through five pairs of trousers a day.

- What might be causing his incontinence and why won't he wear the pads?

Chapter 22

Personal Hygiene, Washing and Bathing

Key messages

- Get to know individual preferences.
- Cultivate the art of pampering!

This is an area which often gives cause for concern and yet with a little insight and some creative thinking most problems can be easily overcome.

Trouble shooting

Try to find out what the person's prior routine and preferences were in matters to do with personal cleanliness. This will involve looking into frequency, times of day and preferred soaps, perfumes etc.

Discussion point

'No way!' You can't expect me to get into that! No, go away! I won't do it. I don't smell, it's not right for me!' And so on it goes for days on end until you realise that he only ever took baths on a Saturday night. Having worked in the fields all week long and being a farm labourer, he could only afford to heat the water once a week and all the family had to take advantage of it. You had a bath on a Saturday so as to be clean for the Sabbath. It was a huge part of the weekly calendar. You could not go to church on Sunday not looking your best.

This is the sort of information you need to find out in order to individualise your approach and in order to understand your clients and avoid avoidable problems!

Did they prefer baths to showers? How often did they bathe and wash? Once a week is the maximum for some people whilst for others one a day is a minimum.

If all else fails and clients with dementia can't tolerate the intrusion of bathing routines, you may have to revise your own standards and compromise.

The frequency of bathing may have to be reduced as it is outweighed by the anxiety it causes the client. Dementia can make the client unaware of the need to bathe; they might have simply forgotten what to do. We are often over sensitive here anyway, so in most cases a simple prompt will suffice. But if not then there is still room for negotiation. When refusal occurs, accept it. Try again later or improvise such as doing bits at a time or just giving frequent, cursory but hygienic strip washes.

Reluctance might be due to the embarrassment of being seen in the nude by strangers or members of the opposite sex. For many people today you still do not undress in public and to be made to do so is quite traumatic. But, equally, a previously easy-going client can be made reluctant by an uncaring and institutional, non-individualised approach.

Independence

Trying to preserve independence, by allowing the person to do as much for themselves as possible, will take you longer. However, it will avoid the commonest cause of problems: the feeling of being interfered with, rushed and not allowed to do things at the pace you want and in the way you want. Given the added elements of confusion and uncertainty that dementia can bring to even the most routine of tasks, it is important that we support the client through the routine rather than de-skill them by taking over and thus worry them by implying that they are no longer capable of something they are probably aware should be easy and straightforward. It must be frightening to have your control over something as intimate as personal hygiene taken away from you. Find out in what order they did things and any individual preferences as regards when and with what. Make sure that everything is ready for them. Do make use of your occupational therapist who can advise on adaptations and equipment which may help to keep the client independent. These might include grab rails which help to get in and out of the bath or on and off the toilet. Raised shower and toilet seats are also a good idea.

Individuality

A little individuality goes a long way. Having talked to relatives and friends about personal preferences, the care assistant is now in a position to make a huge difference to the quality of life of the client (see Exercise 22.1, p.171).

Bath times are also an opportunity for building up relationships with clients, just chatting socially, as opposed to being a care chore or task to be done at the allotted time.

Hair washing, however, can be a frightening experience. Recall the care and patience displayed with babies and young children and recall the trauma of having your own hair washed at a tender age. A mother in a hurry can be a frightening experience, requiring a sharp intake of breath and what seems an eternity to have to hold it. It can be an equally frightening experience for clients with dementia. Pouring water over someone's head can be very frightening for the recipient.

For clients with dementia, the loss of understanding of what might be going on makes it crucial that bath times are taken at a leisurely pace and are skilfully handled. It is not a job; it is not a duty for the unskilled. Making the bath time of a client with dementia a pleasurable event for them is a highly skilled aspect of care. It requires considerable psychological insight and much patience. It needs careful timing, diplomacy and an in-depth knowledge of the individual alongside physical care skills and an awareness of safety issues. Bathing is in fact a perfect example of how a routine aspect of care is taken for granted, alongside those who perform it. Be prepared to stay in the bathroom and allow your client sufficient time.

In residential or nursing homes it is also crucial to ensure privacy so that the client has the opportunity to build up confidence that they will not be disturbed. This rule extends to your care colleagues. If you are indulging your client and using the time to build up a therapeutic relationship then you need privacy. The time will never be special if it is never respected. Make it clear that you cannot be disturbed during a client's bath time.

Other considerations

Toileting, changing clothes, dental care, nail and toe care, hair care and shaving can also present their own particular problems. But again it is tact, diplomacy and a due regard for individuality which will solve most problems.

Health and Social Care National Occupational Standards

This chapter relates to many of the induction and foundation standards but in particular to the following level standards:

Level 2 core units

HSC24 a, b + c Ensure your own actions support the care, protection and well-being of individuals.

Level 2 optional units

HSC27 a, b + c Support individuals in their daily living.
HSC218 a, b + c Support individuals with their personal care needs.
HSC219 a + b Support individuals to manage continence.
HSC246 a + b Maintain a safe and clean environment.

Mental Health Standards

G4.1, 4.2 Enable clients to maintain their personal hygiene and appearance.

Care Homes for Older People: National Minimum Standards

10.1, 10.5, 10.7 These relate to privacy needs of clients.

21.1 to 21.9 These relate to lavatories and washing facilities and require that they are accessible, clearly marked and en suite.

Exercise 22.1

BATHING

- As a staff group just sit quietly and close your eyes.

- Think about your own bath-time routine and think about how occasionally you make it a luxurious event and pamper yourself. Now write on a flip chart all those little things you do to make it a special event.

- The list will be a reflection of a wide range of tastes from getting someone to scrub your back to ensuring complete privacy.

- It is likely to include candles, scents, bubble baths, oils, and even a large glass of whiskey and the football on the radio. Pampering applies to both sexes!

- Now try to come up with a list of preferences for each client and ways in which you can turn what is normally regarded as a routine event into an enjoyable time.

Try to make bathing special and something to be looked forward to.

Chapter 23

Repetition

Key messages

- Recognise the need to offer reassurance and give time.
- Are you spending enough time just socialising with the clients?

For many people with dementia repetition arises simply because short-term memory is severely impaired and they have forgotten they have just asked that question. Such repetition is very 'demanding' in terms of its impact upon our patience. This requires a high degree of tolerance from the carer who should patiently repeat the answer as often as it takes until the client is reassured.

Repetition can also arise out of anxiety or discomfort and is a way of getting attention for some need which the client can't express in a way that we can understand. Try to eliminate all such needs by checking the usual ones (see the 'Hidden meanings and underlying causes' section of Chapter 13). Your reassurance by showing concern will help to diminish this anxiety. Quite often repetition can simply be an expression of the need for human contact and providing short bursts of companionship may be all that is needed to alleviate it.

Within mental health nursing there has been much evidence over the last ten years to suggest that nurse–client interaction is severely diminished. The reasons for this are given as understaffing and the burden of paperwork which accompanies modern nursing practice.

Discussion point

- Discuss whether the working practices you follow are too task oriented as to allow time for meaningful interaction with clients.
- If so, what can you do about it?

Practical tips

- It may be helpful to give generalised responses. These are reassuring for the client and enable the carer not to have to think about a specific response each time. It is particularly useful with severe and constant repetition. A good example would be: 'It's OK, I've taken care of it'. In this way it makes it easier to cope with.

- Validate: ignore the content and focus on the feelings being expressed such as insecurity or fear.

- It may be that in order to cope you sometimes have to 'turn a deaf ear', as long as the client is not too distressed by this lack of response.

- Use cue cards with information written on providing the answer to frequently asked questions.

- Sometimes the repetition is a source of security rather than a sign of insecurity, in much the same way that chanting a mantra can be reassuring and rocking can be a source of comfort. Only by knowing your client well will you be able to judge which it is. If it is comforting to the client then it may need no response from yourself, other than occasional acknowledgement and tolerance of the repetition.

- Share the load and take it in turns to provide the responses and reassurance.

- Is the sufferer bored?

- Try the obvious and check for hearing deficits or faulty hearing aids.

- Where reassurance does not work, and in order to alleviate distress, distraction such as beginning an activity might be useful.

- If all you attempt fails and the person is still anxious, remain with them to provide a reassuring presence.

Health and Social Care National Occupational Standards

This chapter relates to many of the induction and foundation standards but in particular to the following level standards:

Level 2 core units

HSC21 a, b + c Communicate with and complete records for individuals.

Level 2 optional units

HSC27 a, b + c Support individuals in their daily living.
HSC226 a, b + c Support individuals who are distressed.
HSC233 a, b + c Relate to and interact with individuals.

Level 3 core units

HSC31 a, b + c Promote effective communication for and about individuals.

Level 3 optional units

HSC332 a, b + c Support the social, emotional and identity needs of individuals.

HSC369 a, b + c Support individuals with specific communication needs.

Mental Health Standards

J2.1, 2.2 Support individuals when they are distressed.

Chapter 24

Shouting

Key messages
- Ensure clients are sufficiently stimulated and have enough social contact.
- Eliminate common causes of discomfort and anxiety.

Clients may shout and scream or emit a softer but persistent groaning without any apparent cause. There could be many reasons for this which trouble shooting will unearth, such as pain, fear, discomfort, boredom, need for attention etc. But even when we can't find a cause or reason, the person is still experiencing a feeling which causes them distress. This being the case there is a need to validate the feelings and provide comfort. Noise making can be difficult to tolerate in residential settings and it is thus even more important to try to understand the cause rather than just try to eliminate it.

Trouble shooting

- There is often obviously anxiety present and the vocalisations may be a plea for contact, attention and reassurance in the face of a diminishing grasp on reality where less and less is recognisable.

- Try to explore the content for clues which might suggest which unfulfilled need is causing the distress.

- Loneliness and boredom can be sources of distress, so ensure adequate levels of attention, activity and companionship are provided.

- Conversely, over-stimulation or being in a busy environment can give rise to confusion and feelings of being overwhelmed and not understanding. A reaction to this might be to scream.

- Eliminate physical causes of distress, especially pain and discomfort. Obvious needs such as toileting, hunger and thirst should be checked.

- Check hearing and hearing aids.

- Check that the client's environment is comfortable and not too hot or cold.

- Fear can often be a cause of shouting, especially during the night when clients may feel even more alone.

- If the person is calling out for someone from their past, validate the feelings and explore that past with them.

- If all else fails try using distraction to minimise their distress.

Discussion point

Pauline has severe dementia and has to have a lot of assistance with many things. She has little language ability and carers can make no sense of her utterances. She is found one day curled up in a ball on the floor, rocking slowly and crying out loudly. She is in tears.

What might be the problem here and how would you handle the situation?

Health and Social Care National Occupational Standards

This chapter relates to many of the induction and foundation standards but in particular to the following level standards:

Level 2 core units

HSC21 a, b + c Communicate with and complete records for individuals.

Level 2 optional units

HSC27 a, b + c Support individuals in their daily living.
HSC226 a, b + c Support individuals who are distressed.
HSC233 a, b + c Relate to and interact with individuals.

Level 3 core units

HSC31 a, b + c Promote effective communication for and about individuals.

Level 3 optional units

HSC332 a, b + c Support the social, emotional and identity needs of individuals.
HSC369 a, b + c Support individuals with specific communication needs.

Mental Health Standards

A4.1, 4.2 Promote effective communication and relationships.
A5.1, 5.2 Promote effective communication and relationships with people who are troubled or distressed.
J2.1, 2.2 Support individuals when they are distressed.

Exercise 24.1

VISITOR STRESS AND INSIGHT

Alan is a happy client who especially enjoys the visits of his daughter and grand-children. However, the daughter is always in a hurry and seldom stops for more than half an hour. After every visit and hurried departure, Alan stares out of the window then paces up and down shouting. No one can make out what he is saying and it usually only lasts about half an hour, but it is distressing for Alan and for the other residents. This is an example with an obvious cause.

How would you handle it at the time and what might you be able to do to reduce its recurrence?

Chapter 25

Sleep Disturbance

Key messages

- Use the trouble shooting process to elicit the cause.
- Be aware of the client's previous sleep patterns.

It is common for dementia sufferers to be somewhat restless during the night from time to time and this can be problematic in a nursing home or residential setting. Disorientation in time is a major effect of dementia and it can lead people to think in the middle of the night that it is morning and time to get up and go to work. The onset of darkness has also been an important part of many people's lives signifying time to go home, go to work, to put the kids to bed, to go out. These habits die hard. It is also a busy time in an institutional setting with bedding routines often being finished before the night staff come on duty. This strict adherence to routine may in itself cause many problems by eroding any individual approach to evening care.

> **Discussion point**
> Consider the night-time routine in your home. Does it cater for individual needs and clients' pre-institutional habits?

Trouble shooting

- Is the client looking for the toilet?

- Are they sleeping too much during the day?

- Are they going to bed too early?

- Is the institutional routine too rigid as to allow them to follow their own lifelong night-time/bedtime and sleeping routine?

- Having woken up in the middle of the night, are they scared as to where they are, confused and in need of reassurance? Use a night light to provide some reassurance should they awake in the night.

- Do they think it is time to get up?

- Does the routine fit in with their past? Were they shift workers and early starters? Do they think they are going to work?

- Increase physical activity levels during the day time so that people are tired at night time. If clients are left sitting all day long doing nothing, dozing in a chair, then we cannot expect them to sleep all night.

- Consider the possibility that people are over-medicated to the degree that they are inactive during the day and thus less in need of sleep.

- Are they uncomfortable? Discomfort should be eliminated. Is the bed appropriate for the client? Is the room too hot or cold?

- Make sure clients do not go to bed hungry.

- If the client has difficulties getting to sleep, try relaxing music and aromatherapy or massage. A nice warm, scented bath will do no harm.

- Check for physical discomfort, such as pain or constipation.

- Check whether the restlessness could be caused by the side effects of medication.

Health and Social Care National Occupational Standards

This chapter relates to many of the induction and foundation standards but in particular to the following level standards:

Level 2 core units

HSC21 a, b + c Communicate with and complete records for individuals.

Level 2 optional units

HSC27 a, b + c Support individuals in their daily living.
HSC216 a, b Help address the physical comfort needs of individuals.
HSC226 a, b + c Support individuals who are distressed.
HSC233 a, b + c Relate to and interact with individuals.

Level 3 core units

HSC35 a, b + c Promote choice, well-being and the protection of all individuals.

Chapter 26

Withdrawal and Non-Communication

Key messages
- Give clients attention, as often they cannot ask for it or initiate it.
- Check for depression as this is a common accompaniment to dementia.

'He just used to sit there all day and never talk.'

'He never acknowledges me, never seems to want to talk.'

These are common sentiments from carers describing the loneliness they felt while caring for their spouses at home. The withdrawal and lack of communication carers often experience from their loved ones can be psychologically draining. The sense of isolation for the carer can be intolerable. Clients suffering dementia often try to withdraw from a world that makes little sense to them. Doing so may be a source of comfort for the client: if you do not interact with the world you cannot experience not understanding it; if you do not interact you do not experience failure, bewilderment and sadness. Better to withdraw into your own world.

> ### Discussion point
> A wife who brought her husband in for respite told you that she was miserable because her husband no longer spoke to her. What advice could you give her?

Trouble shooting

- *Attention/awareness* – Clients may be too afraid of getting things wrong or muddling words to dare speak. They may also often lose track of what is being said and so choose to withdraw from communicating.

- *Cuddles* – The very confused and those lacking in any short-term memory can often get upset and can isolate themselves, but they still know what a cuddle is, and this should be used as a regular inclusion exercise and stress reduction tool.

- *Sensory deprivation* – Check the clients for sensory deprivation. If one of their senses is declining, concentrate on another. If sight and hearing are poor then touch becomes even more important. Often lack of communication is due to the client not understanding our question because we do not slow down enough for them.

- *Body language* – This is still understood by people with dementia, so use it carefully. You can convey many important messages via gesture, smile and facial expression. Be aware also of maintaining personal space. Be mindful, also, of how you say things, as this can convey affection and trust.

- *Depression* – This is common in dementia and often goes under-reported; clients may have insight into diminishing mental powers and generalised sadness at their failing abilities. When people with dementia do get depressed they often withdraw into the relative safety of non-communication. Check the client's appetite and sleep patterns and if in doubt ask for a psychiatric opinion, as depression can be hard to recognise and is often overlooked.

- *Short bursts* – The attention span of people with dementia is short so keep communications short and simple. Activity can draw people out of their shells but again it needs to be in short bursts.

Health and Social Care National Occupational Standards

This chapter relates to many of the induction and foundation standards but in particular to the following level standards:

Level 2 core units

HSC21 a, b + c Communicate with and complete records for individuals.

Level 2 optional units

HSC27 a, b + c Support individuals in their daily living.
HSC210 a, b + c Support individuals to access and participate in recreational activities.
HSC226 a, b + c Support individuals who are distressed.
HSC233 a, b + c Relate to and interact with individuals.

Level 3 core units

HSC31 a, b + c Promote effective communication for and about individuals.

Level 3 optional units

HSC332 a, b + c Support the social, emotional and identity needs of individuals.

HSC369 a, b + c Support individuals with specific communication needs.

Chapter 27

Normalisation and Inclusion

Key messages

- It is the ordinary 'humdrum' aspects of everyday life in which we need to include clients.
- Part of being normal includes having a role in the household.

This section relates to making life as near normal as possible given the constraints of living in a residential or nursing home. The key to achieving this is by involving clients in as many aspects of their lives as possible and giving them back responsibilities and roles. Institutional care strips away much responsibility for looking after yourself – there is no need to shop, budget, cook, launder, etc. But by keeping people involved in these sorts of outwardly mundane and very domestic tasks you are helping them to retain a sense of control over their own lives. Below are some thoughts and ideas for fostering normalisation and inclusion.

Rooms

How normal are your clients' rooms? Think about the rooms in your own house and how much personal 'stuff' you have littered about the place, possessions and assorted mementos etc. Are all your clients' rooms similar? If so, why? Take the time with colleagues to undertake an audit one day. Tour all your clients' rooms and write down what it is about each one which makes it personal to that client. Then get together and discuss how you can change the room to reflect the values and interests of the client even more. It is about making the leap from 'This is the room where Shelley sleeps' to 'This is Shelley's room'. Ask for help from relatives to get a picture of how the client might like their room if they are not capable of telling you. Did they like clutter, were they more minimalist or just tidy? What personal items can be used to personalise their room? Suggestions are: their favourite armchair; pictures of their hobbies, home town and family or favourite holiday spots; photographs and personal objects or treasured possessions such as souvenirs from holidays – all these will help to personalise the room. These can be displayed on bookshelves. The room should be such that the client would want to bring visitors in and entertain them. We all have different preferences for decoration too, so try and find out what the client's own choice of décor would be and whether you could do anything to achieve it.

Celebrations

It is normal to recognise events in life with celebrations and we all have our own ways of doing this. Try to find out what your client's preferred ways of celebrating were: did they enjoy a big party or did they prefer a meal out or a small family affair? Then list the significant events in your client's life and ensure that they get marked with an appropriate celebration.

Parties

Make excuses for parties in nursing and residential homes. These provide excellent opportunities for social interaction and stimulation. Celebrate anything! Parties are also an excuse for much other activity such as food preparation, baking, decorating the room, choosing the music, getting dressed up, etc. An informal atmosphere at a party can be a good opportunity to draw in the quieter members of the community and help them to feel more involved and belonging.

Outside involvement

How many of your clients retain links with the outside world? How often do they go out of the building? The more your clients do of either of these, then the nearer they are to normal life. Often clients will have had strong community-based associations such as with churches and through membership of hobby-related organisations. With the help of friends and relatives, clients should be facilitated to retain such links. If clients can't go out then the outside world should be encouraged to come to them. Thus a group of friends from the church could come to visit and hold a short service or prayer meeting. Similarly friends from the club could come and hold a meeting and create the opportunity to have a few drinks together. The football fan should be taken to the match and the bird watcher to the marshes.

It is often the case that a move to residential care signals the end of day centre attendance. This is short sighted. Such a time is likely to be one whereby the person needs to retain outside links, not have them curtailed.

Possessions

A big part of normal life and a great source of comfort to most of us is the simple fact of being surrounded by treasured and personal possessions. All too often in institutions one sees very little physical evidence of the client or their previous life through their possessions. Bedrooms all tend to look very similar apart from the odd photograph. Carers need to positively encourage clients to retain as many personal possessions as possible. Many are very small but hugely valuable and can easily be kept in a box or drawer. Others can be placed in a cabinet or on shelves. But people should also be encouraged to bring with them bigger items, such as a favourite chair, cabinet or chest of drawers. Often personal collections are lost in the transition to care and this needs to be carefully guarded against. The reminiscence possibilities of such possessions are many and doubly important in dementia care.

Choices

Making choices is something we take for granted, but is often denied clients in institutions, even more so if they suffer a dementia. Part of the cause of this is the wrong opinion that people with dementia can't choose and don't care. This is blatantly not true. But how often do we offer obvious choices such as what to eat, for example? How can you provide choices for your clients at mealtimes? What changes can be made to mealtime routines to allow more choice in what to eat, when to eat and where to eat? We also choose, frequently, to have a quick snack or a cup of tea. How often do we offer this choice to our clients? Examine the ways in which you can introduce the opportunity to make choices into your clients' lives.

Dressing is another obvious example of an area which could offer many choices. We should be striving to help people look the way they did before they became ill. In doing so carers need to pay attention to style and make-up etc. and offer a range of choices. This has the added bonus of giving people a little pampering and helping them feel good about the way they look. You are helping them to realise that they matter. You will need to pay attention to communication skills when offering choices. Remember to keep things simple, which may mean narrowing down the choice. Thus 'Would you like a biscuit, Lorna' and offering her the tin to choose from is far more empowering than saying, 'OK Lorna, do you want a Bourbon, a digestive or a custard cream?' or just giving her a biscuit of your choosing.

Normal life

When we talk about activities with clients we invariably think of art and craft, singalongs, bingo and the like. Yet by far the most important activities are those normal everyday things we take for granted and which might seem rather boring and humdrum. Being involved in everyday life gives us a role, credibility and a sense of being involved in our own lives rather than having everything done for us. Being denied a part in looking after yourself can be very depressing.

It is a blow to self-esteem when you are no longer needed to meet your own requirements. In dementia we often have to take over responsibility for certain tasks, but we do not have to exclude the client and involvement in everyday tasks such as doing the laundry or washing the car can be very fulfilling for clients.

Discussion point

This is possibly the most important question and exercise in the book as far as making a difference to clients is concerned.

- What opportunities can you think of for including your clients in ordinary life tasks?

- Think about ways in which the running of the home or staff routines can be altered to help this to happen.

Jacki Pritchard (2003) came up with a clear list of questions asking whether service users had the right to do certain things and it is worth considering some of them here, slightly adapted to suit clients with a dementia, and including everyday activity related to normal life.

Can our clients – or do our clients – have the opportunity to:

- shop for their clothes

- go out for a walk when they want

- have an alcoholic drink

- have sex

- choose what to eat and wear

- bathe when they want and refuse when they want

- go to bed when they want

- get up when they want

- wash up

- put the rubbish out

- feed the cat

- fill the car up

- clean the house

- paint the fence

- change the bulb

- go to the supermarket

- walk the dog

- fetch the papers

- nip out for a pint of milk

- change the bed?

This list could go on and on. As a staff team think about ways in which you could include your dementia sufferers in the ordinary but fulfilling tasks of life.

Conclusion

People with dementia have the right to live as near normal an existence as possible. They have a right to individualised care, meaningful activity and participation in everyday life. Other rights are having choices, privacy, personal possessions, dignity and some control over their existence. Whilst normalisation is a valid goal, people with dementia also require specialist care. However, specialist care homes have a duty to work towards deinstitutionalisation. This becomes political in the sense that many carers work in private homes and the bulk of long-term dementia care exists today within this commercial sphere. Often the need to make a profit can detract from the desire to provide quality care. Hotel aspects of care such as décor, furniture and food are frequently very good, but activity levels are often low. This is a form of abuse, as the explicit mental health and stimulation needs of clients are not being met. Carers in these environments have a duty to lobby for extra resources to foster normalisation and to blow the whistle on neglect of human rights.

Health and Social Care National Occupational Standards

This chapter relates to many of the induction and foundation standards but in particular to the following level standards:

Level 2 core units

HSC21b Listen to and respond to individuals' questions and concerns.
HSC24a Relate to and support individuals in the way they choose.
HSC27 a, b + c Support individuals in their daily living.
HSC210 a, b + c Support individuals to access and participate in recreational activities.
HSC211 a, b + c Support individuals to take part in developmental activities.
HSC218 a, b + c Support individuals with their personal care needs.

Level 2 optional units

HSC233 a + b Relate to and interact with individuals.
HSC234 a + b Ensure your own actions support the equality, diversity, rights and responsibilities of individuals.

Level 3 core units

> HSC33 a + b Reflect on and develop your practice.
>
> HSC35 a + b Promote choice and independence and respect the diversity and difference of individuals.

Level 3 optional units

> HSC330 a, b + c Support individuals to access and use services and facilities.
>
> HSC332 a, b + c Support the social, emotional and identity needs of the individual.
>
> HSC334 a, b + c Provide a home and family environment for individuals.
>
> HSC350 a, b + c Recognise, respect and support the spiritual well-being of individuals.
>
> HSC3111 a + b Promote equality, diversity, rights and responsibilities of individuals.
>
> HSC3116 a, b + c Contribute to promoting a culture that values and respects the diversity of individuals.

Level 4 core units

> HSC43 a + b Take responsibility for the continuing professional development of self and others.

Level 4 optional units

> HSC414 Assess individual needs and preferences.

Mental Health Standards

> G11.1, 11.2, 11.3 Promote the social inclusion of people with mental health needs.
>
> G12.1, 12.2 Represent individuals' interests when they are not able to do so themselves.
>
> H4.1, 4.2 Support people in relation to personal and social interactions and environmental factors.
>
> M3.1, 3.2, 3.3 Contribute to developing and maintaining cultures and strategies in which people are respected and valued as individuals.

Care Homes for Older People: National Minimum Standards

> 7.1 to 7.6 These standards relate to an individualised plan of care based on a comprehensive assessment.
>
> 10.3 Service users wear their own clothes at all times.
>
> 14.1 to 14.5 These standards relate to allowing clients to exercise choice and control over their lives.

Further reading and references

Pritchard, J. (2003) *Training Manual for Working with Older People in Residential and Day Care Settings.* London: Jessica Kingsley Publishers.

Redfern, S. (1997) 'Supporting residents in long stay settings.' In I. Norman and S. Redfern (eds) *Mental Health Care for Elderly People.* Edinburgh: Churchill Livingstone.

Exercise 27.1

POSSESSIONS

- You wake up in the middle of the night and smell smoke. It is your worst nightmare: the house is on fire.

- There is precious little time to get out of the building safely. But you clutch at a small suitcase and desperately rush to gather your most treasured possessions.

- You only have time to save five things. What will they be?

- Do this exercise with colleagues and share your lists afterwards.

- Explain to each other why the objects mean so much to you.

- Now on a flip chart write down the names of all your clients and besides each one write down the five things you think they would have saved.

- If you can't think of them discuss how you could get to know what they might be.

You will have to refer to relatives and friends. Once you get the list, consider how you might go about obtaining the items for the client.

Chapter 28
Care Planning

Key message

Care is not static. Assessment is an ongoing process with care being constantly evaluated and altered to changing circumstances and needs.

One of the things we can learn from nursing care in hospital settings is the importance and usefulness of care plans. The 'nursing process', as it is known, involves a cyclical awareness of the client's needs. It involves four stages, namely assessment, planning, implementation and evaluation. After the evaluation stage, you reassess and go around again. In this way the client's needs are constantly being monitored and the care given adjusted accordingly (see Figure 28.1).

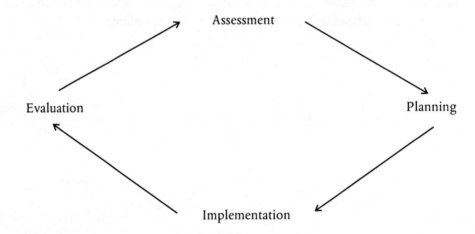

Figure 28.1 The nursing process

The assessment is a crucial stage because if you get the assessment of the client's needs wrong then you will be providing care which does not meet the client's needs. It is important therefore that you have a good assessment tool. Chapter 6 on client history indicates areas which a good assessment should cover, alongside physical care needs and any moving and handling or other special instructions.

To achieve a client centred assessment, it is good practice to include the client as much as possible; where this is not possible, the relatives and friends of the client should be involved.

The care plan based on such an assessment outlines the individual care needed by each person. Treating each client as an individual is important, as the alternative is strict adherence to routines which do not suit everybody and an erosion of individuality. It is often easy in care settings to lose the sense that all clients are unique individuals.

A good care plan will look at all aspects of a person's life, catering for their physical, spiritual, social and psychological needs.

> In Tony's care plan it is stated that he needs a milky coffee with digestive biscuits for supper at 10.30 every night. It also states that it is imperative that he does not miss any Arsenal game on the television. He watches the church service on the television on a Sunday morning and loves wildlife programmes. He loved walking in the Scottish hills and has a drop of scotch every Friday and Saturday night. Two drops if Arsenal lose, three if they win.

The planning stage of the care plan process is crucial also because here you state exactly what you are going to do to address the need you have identified. There is absolutely no point in having a care plan if it does not get to the soul of the client. The comments above about drops of scotch might appear flippant but they are the important detail which is so often ignored. Without these it might be anybody's care plan and not Tony's. Nursing care plans tend to be illness related and physically oriented out of necessity. However, nursing-home care plans should be much more personal statements about individual preferences. We should regard the person as a tenant not a client: this is their home, not just their temporary residence as in a hospital situation.

The care plan is not just a list if the client's likes and dislikes, it should also be an indicator of how the client's strengths and skills can be utilised and maintained.

Monthly appraisal

Care plans need to be regularly reviewed to take into account any changes in care needs. Each hand-over between shifts is an opportunity to review care, but to take the process further staff should hold monthly care plan reviews with their clients. Each client should have a key worker whose responsibility this is. The role of the key worker in nursing and residential settings is to ensure that the client gets maximum satisfaction and enjoyment out of life. In institutions it is not the décor or quality of the food which makes the most difference to clients' lives, it is the quality of relationships they have and the activity and stimulation they receive, the feeling of belonging and of being valued. These are the issues which should be central to a care plan, over and above more basic physical needs.

Health and Social Care National Occupational Standards

This chapter relates to many of the induction and foundation standards but in particular to the following level standards:

Level 2 core units

HSC21d Access and update records and reports.

Level 2 optional units

HSC25 a, b + c Carry out and provide feedback on specific plan of care activities.
HSC224 a, b + c Observe, monitor and record the conditions of individuals.

Level 3 optional units

HSC328 a, b + c Contribute to care planning and review.
HSC368a Identify, with individuals, the needs and preferences they want you to present.
HSC368b Act with and on behalf of individuals, according to their needs and wishes.

Level 4 optional units

HSC416 a, b + c Develop, implement and review care plans with individuals.

Mental Health Standards

C2.1, 2.2, 2.3, 2.4 Develop, implement and review programmes of support for carers and families.
D4.1 Identify individuals' needs and circumstances.
E1.1, 1.2, 1.3, 1.4 Contribute to the development, provision and review of care programmes.

Care Homes for Older People: National Minimum Standards

7.1 to 7.6 These standards relate to service users having a plan of care relating to their health, personal and social care needs and in which the service user is involved. Such plans should be reviewed monthly.

Chapter 29

Physical Care

Key message

Clients often can't communicate to us what ails them so carers need to be very proactive in recognising signs of discomfort.

Loss of self-care skills and reduced cognitive function renders our clients vulnerable to physical complications as they may not be able to look after themselves or recognise the risk that changes in environmental conditions bring. Alongside this is a loss of ability to communicate what is wrong and, because of this, problems can escalate before carers become aware of them.

Skin care

The immobile older person has an increased risk of problems in regard to skin breaking down. In the later stages of a dementia pressure sores are common and the added complication of incontinence where acidic urine is in frequent contact with the skin can cause severe problems. The pressure sore arises from the skin being compressed and the blood supply being curtailed. This denies the skin oxygen, nutrients and fluids and so it breaks down. It is frequently a problem for those who are immobile and bedridden as they cannot shift their weight from area to area.

Sufferers who are incontinent can wear pads that collect the urine and faeces, but they must be frequently changed and high standards of skin care must be given, with regular washing and the use of barrier creams to prevent sores and skin breakdown. It is also important that the person has an adequate fluid intake to prevent tissue breakdown. It is tempting to reduce the fluid intake of sufferers who are incontinent but this is counter-productive. Similarly, long periods of inactivity are to be avoided. A programme of short walks or exercise should be care planned for those at greatest risk. If, in the later stages, this is not possible, then consideration should be given to pressure-relieving cushions and mattresses.

Teeth

It is important to maintain oral care as gum and tooth problems can be very painful. Oral hygiene should be a part of normal daily care with carers giving clients reminders or helping with brushing or denture care. This provides an opportunity to check for problems on a regular basis. Arguably each client should be seen by a dentist at least once a year. Such visits can be distressing and much reassurance will be required. It might be possible for a dentist to visit the care home as this would help to reduce the trauma.

Temperature regulation

In the later stages of dementia the person may not be able to recognise that it is too cold or too hot. You may have to ensure that they are adequately clothed for the prevailing weather conditions. When the person with advanced dementia gets cold they do not counter this with exercise to generate heat as the rest of us might. They may also not recognise the need to put on extra clothing or be able to do this. Carers need to spot this deficit and be proactive in ensuring that their clients are comfortable in relation to the surrounding temperature.

We often take this need for granted, and being warm is one of the most basic of human needs; however, in dementia the ability to control this is often lost. Simple measures, such as ensuring that the client is not sitting in a draught, will go a long way towards enhancing their quality of life. Similarly, be aware of the dangers of sitting in the sun too long or of leaving open a window in the bathroom.

Diet

A good healthy diet is crucial in dementia. The client has enough problems without adding to them. Too few vitamins and other essentials can lead to an increase in confusion and susceptibility to infections and colds. Creativity and skilful use of supplements are the key to maintaining nutrition in clients who insist upon their own regimes. There is little point in forcing an issue when the client is beyond rational argument. Once again the importance of a good therapeutic relationship is the key to success. It is particularly important that the person has a good fluid intake, takes regular exercise and generally has a good supply of vegetables, fruit and cereals.

Constipation

Constipation is linked to nutrition and is one of the commonest causes of confusion amongst older people, especially those who are not very mobile. A preventative measure for constipation is ensuring that clients get plenty of exercise. This also helps clients overcome sleep problems. Yet activity is an area which many nursing and residential homes still fall behind on. Many would deny this but if you eliminate the activity organiser concentrating on the most able, then you are drawn into the conclusion that there is still much to be done here.

The senses

The eyes and ears of dementia sufferers should be checked on a regular basis. This is especially important in the light of the communication difficulties dementia can bring. A hearing aid might help those with poor hearing, but it might be difficult for the person with dementia to get used to it. If not used properly an aid could well cause more distress than good. If this is the case you will have to rely upon your own communication skills. Make sure there are no distractions such as a loud television. Get the person's attention, perhaps by touching them on the arm. Face them and speak slowly but clearly.

Clients who wear glasses can often forget to use them and will need to be reminded at times. Similarly carers need to ensure that glasses are clean. If their vision is failing it might be equally difficult for the person with dementia to get used to wearing spectacles. Again it could cause more distress than benefit. However, sight tests are important for highlighting treatable conditions such as glaucoma or cataracts.

Feet

Feet need to be cared for and should be checked once a week as part of the routine. Seek advice from a chiropodist as to the best way to cut toenails. You need to be aware of the possibility of ingrowing toenails which can be very painful. Any unusual redness or swelling which persists should be reported to the GP. As a general rule try to keep feet clean and dry.

Annual health check

Remember that anyone over 75 is entitled to an annual health check. Insist that your clients get theirs and insist that it is thorough. 'Insist' is not too strong a word here as there is much evidence to suggest that the needs of dementia sufferers are all too often ignored by primary care services. Research suggests that GPs frequently overlook the needs of the dementia client with regard to both onward referral for a psychiatric opinion and the thorough assessment of physical needs.

Health and Social Care National Occupational Standards

This chapter relates to many of the induction and foundation standards but in particular to the following level standards:

Level 2 core units

> HSC24 a, b + c Ensure your own actions support the care, protection and well-being of individuals.

Level 2 optional units

> HSC215 a + b Help individuals to keep mobile.
>
> HSC216 a + b Help address the physical comfort needs of the individual.
>
> HSC217 a + b Undertake agreed pressure area care.
>
> HSC220 a + b Maintain the feet of individuals who have been assessed as requiring help with general foot care.
>
> HSC225 a + b Support individuals to undertake and monitor their own health care.
>
> HSC228a Contribute to group care that supports the physical, social and emotional needs of the group and its members.
>
> HSC246 a + b Maintain a safe and clean environment.

Level 3 optional units

> HSC358 a, b + c Identify the individual at risk of skin breakdown and undertake the appropriate risk assessment.
>
> HSC364 a, b + c Identify the physical health needs of individuals with mental health problems.
>
> HSC3103 a, b + c Contribute to raising awareness of health issues.

Mental Health Standards

> D5.1, 5.2 Identify the physical health needs of individuals with mental health needs.
>
> F7.1, 7.2 Support people with mental health needs to improve their physical health and well-being.

Care Homes for Older People: National Minimum Standards

> 8.1 to 8.13 These standards all focus on ensuring that service users' health care needs are fully met.
>
> 10.1, 10.5, 10.7 These relate to privacy needs of clients.
>
> 21.1 to 21.9 These relate to lavatories and washing facilities and require that they are accessible, clearly marked and ensuite.

Further reading and references

Adams, T. and Manthorpe, J. (2003) *Dementia Care*. London: Arnold.

Medcof, J. and Roth, J. (eds) (1979) *Approaches to Psychology*. Milton Keynes: Open University Press. Chapter 7, 'The humanistic approach', gives a good overview of Maslow and his theory of the hierarchy of needs.

Exercise 29.1
HIERARCHY OF NEEDS

Read up about Abraham Maslow (Medcof and Roth 1979) and his concept of the hierarchy of needs. Then ask yourself whether your assessments and care plans cater for the lower- and higher-order needs as explained by Maslow.

Chapter 30

The Care Environment

Key message
We need to adapt buildings and routines to suit the clients not the clients to suit our routines.

As carers we need to look at the care environment. We can't often change the actual structure of the building, but we can change the way we use it. We need to examine how we can adapt it to help the clients rather than hinder them (see Exercise 30.1, p.202). Ideas will include the following:

- An area which can be used for shared activity, such as craft work.

- An area which lends itself to socialising and parties.

- Areas which are private or semi-private for individuals to use.

- Making it easy for clients to find their way around.

- Ensuring that the lighting is adequate. Are there any dark areas?

- Recreating the past. Clients with dementia are often fixed in a past time: how does the environment mirror that time in order to make them feel at home? If you lived and grew up in the 1940s and that is what you feel is the period now, how does the care home help you to feel at home? Is there too much modern furniture? Many of those with dementia have no recollection of living in the modern world and we need to create homely environments with the characteristics of the client's previous homes – 1940s furniture, ornaments and music etc.

- Ensuring that the furniture is comfortable and supportive. Are the chairs easy to get in and out of?

- Thinking about how willing we are to let clients bring their own furniture into the care home.

- The door to the toilet being identifiable and easy to find. If clients can't recognise it then it might be that a label has to be placed on the door. Better still, place a picture of a toilet on the door to aid recognition. This might be regarded as institutionalising but it is worth it to preserve independence.

- Recognisable bedrooms. Many clients' bedrooms are in corridors where all the rooms look alike. This can easily be resolved by putting the client's name and photograph and other personal information or mementos on the door. This is a form of reminiscence as well as an aid to identity and orientation. You could pin a picture of a Labrador dog or a doll on the door. Experiment with different cues and clues, to find something that the person can link between that door and themselves.

- Safety features can be incorporated into buildings: wooden grill covers can be placed over radiators, windows can be installed which only open a little way and you should ensure the hot water does not exceed a safe temperature.

- Provision for clients to wander in safety without staff having to constantly worry about their whereabouts.

- Gardens should be considered also. These ought to be places where the client can wander in safety, but without feeling locked in or restricted. Careful design and planting can achieve this effect and many distractions, apart from plants, can be incorporated into a garden – statues, water features and seats, for example.

- Check that the temperature is at the right level, not too hot or too chilly. Are there any obvious draughts? You don't necessarily feel them if you are a busy carer, so try sitting for a while, now and again, in lots of different areas, to check for this.

- Does the care home look like an institution?

- Does the lounge look like your mother's sitting room or a doctor's waiting room? Is there a fireplace with a mantelpiece, clock, photo, pipe rack, candle and other paraphernalia? Sit in it for a couple of hours, don't read or talk to your colleagues, just soak up the feeling the room gives off. Discuss your findings and thoughts with your colleagues. Check the layout of the furniture and arrange it in different groups as opposed to lines or around the outside of the room. What homely features and fittings can be used?

- Think about how the bathroom stands up to scrutiny? Is it instantly institutional or does it have a homely and old-fashioned feel? If not, how can this be accomplished? As with the living room this desire to camouflage the institutional aspects must be in keeping with allowing clients to remain independent. This latter goal often necessitates the use of equipment such as hoists, grab rails and other aids. The independence must always come first, but it is possible to achieve a blend and make even a heavily adapted environment age appropriate, homely and 'normal'.

- Corridors are often bleak spaces but with careful adaptation they can become stimulating places in which to wander. How can you make them interesting and safe? What can you put in them to look at and touch and make people want to linger there and enjoy being in them?

Noise: A special case

This is an often overlooked, but very invasive, aspect of communal life. How often have you walked into an institutional lounge to find the television blaring out but nobody watching it? Similarly, radios are left playing, often to suit the needs of staff members, and often playing a kind of music not likely to be appreciated by the clients. Using the television or radio as background noise is no subStitute for shared activity or conversation and contact. Add to this the hustle and bustle of caring and the cleaning and domestic routine of the care home and it can all become quite a disturbance. This can be anxiety provoking and very stressful for clients. Too much noise will add to a sense of confusion and bewilderment.

Discussion point

- What are the noise levels in your care home like?
- Are televisions and radios used for the benefit of staff?
- How can the noise be managed so that it does not cause distress?

Health and Social Care National Occupational Standards

This chapter relates to many of the induction and foundation standards but in particular to the following level standards:

Level 3 core units

HSC35a Develop supportive relationships that promote choice and independence.

Level 3 optional units

HSC334 a, b + c Provide a home and family environment for individuals.

Care Homes for Older People: National Minimum Standards

10.1 to 10.7 These standards relate to issues of privacy and maintenance of dignity.

19.1 to 19.6 These relate to a safe environment.

20.1 to 20.7 These relate to shared facilities and communal areas. There is an emphasis on safety and comfort.

21.1 to 21.9 These relate to washing and lavatory facilities with an emphasis on privacy and ease of use.

22.1 to 22.8 These relate to adaptations and equipment which must be user friendly and encourage independence.

23.1 to 23.10 These relate to the space requirements of individual accommodation.

24.1 to 24.8 These relate to the furniture and fittings within individual accommodation. They lay down minimum requirements for comfort, privacy and safety.

25.1 to 25.8 These relate to standards for heating and lighting, again with an emphasis on safety and comfort.

26.1 to 26.9 These relate to standards of cleanliness and hygiene.

✓

Exercise 30.1

ENVIRONMENTAL CHANGE

- Think about the care home you work in and the needs of people with dementia.

- What aspects of the *environment* can have an impact upon a client's well being?

Just take two aspects of dementia, the fact that clients have poor memory and the fact that they can suffer high levels of stress.

- What aspects of the environment have a negative impact upon these?

- What can be done about it?

Chapter 31

Depression and Dementia

Key messages

- Depression is a common accompaniment to dementia and is often overlooked.
- Depression can and should be treated.

Depression in dementia is quite common but often unrecognised. If you think about the early stages of dementia when the sufferer still has some insight, then the realisation that you are losing your mind, memory and ability to think, the sense of loss of control over your own mind must be very traumatic. Anyone would be depressed at this realisation. Indeed, it is difficult for the rest of us to appreciate just how frightening this must be. Added to this is the humiliation of others having to guide and direct you to perform even the most basic of tasks. The loss of self-esteem must be enormous and it is easy to see why so many dementia sufferers withdraw from social contact in the early stages. It is to protect them from the humiliation of others realising they can no longer look after themselves.

Depression

Everybody experiences periods of low mood and despair, it is part of life. But when that despair deepens and persists over time, it is a sign of clinical depression. The symptoms are things we all suffer from time to time – low mood, feelings of hopelessness, poor appetite, inability to sleep, anxiety, loss of interest in hobbies, low self-esteem, withdrawal, poor concentration and memory, physical slowing down or, perversely, agitation. While depression causes a chemical imbalance in the brain, it can nearly always be traced back to trigger events in the person's life. Isolation and loneliness are common precursors of depression as is bereavement and loss. The sufferer of dementia can feel much loss, an overwhelming sense of isolation and a frightening loss of control. People with dementia therefore are just as likely to become depressed as a result of adverse life events as are people without a dementia, if not more so.

> **Discussion point**
>
> - Discuss the losses a person diagnosed with dementia might be faced with.
> - Think about the early stages and the later stages and about the whole range of physical, social and psychological changes and losses occurring.

As the dementia progresses the gradual loss of ability, continual exposure to failure and deepening sense of bewilderment and anxiety, if not fear, will all encourage depression. In the later stages of dementia, boredom and inactivity can also contribute.

The coexistence of depression alongside dementia is entirely understandable and must be profoundly disabling. In the early stages, as well as a sense of loss and failure of ability there is also the worry of what the future holds and how you will cope. Such a combination of both depression and dementia is likely to make the appearance of the dementia worse, with greater memory loss and confusion, more isolation and even agitation. It will also have the effect of reducing the already diminished capacity for self-care.

Dementia or depression

Depression in dementia can be difficult to diagnose because the signs and symptoms of depression are similar to the early stages of dementia: poor concentration, poor memory, low intelligence test scores and withdrawal. All of these can be indications of both depression and dementia.

While the depressed person has no real memory loss or cognitive impairment they will perform poorly in tests because the depression has reduced their powers of concentration and motivation. When faced with a particular task, the person with dementia will often have a go and persevere whilst the person with depression will often not even try or will give up easily because they have no motivation. The person with depression is more likely to complain about their poor memory and concentration than the person with dementia, who may well try to cover it up. Such a depression is often termed 'depressive pseudo dementia' because it so closely resembles the symptoms of dementia.

There are other ways of telling the two apart. Depression is often worse in the morning. The thoughts of the depressed person are negative and sad while those of the dementia sufferer may not be so consistent or negative but will display some repetition. The person with dementia might give you incorrect answers to questions whereas the person with depression will tell you they do not know or cannot be bothered to think about it. On formal testing the person with depression will tend to give up easily and make little effort while the person with dementia will try hard but perform poorly.

Relocation

Relocation can be a traumatic event for any of us and research shows that rates of depression in nursing and residential homes are often very much higher than in those living at home. The impact of such a relocation into institutional care is likely to be a major trigger factor for depression and great care must be taken to ensure that the move does not induce this.

Discussion point
How can a relocation be managed to ensure that the risk of depression is minimised?

Antidepressants

These will restore the chemical imbalance in the brain, but can often take over three weeks to work and must be taken for at least six months to guard against the possibility of a relapse. There are different kinds of antidepressant and it is often a matter of finding one which suits each individual client.

Listening

Taking the time to be with and listen to the concerns of the person with dementia who is also depressed is crucial. This will help to validate their feelings and show that others are concerned. This will in turn help to boost their sense of self-worth. Often depressed people feel unworthy of the attention of others and it is important to combat this by demonstrating concern and pointing out their value.

Person centred approach

Where depression and dementia coexist a basic person centred care approach is needed. This will mirror good care for any client with depression. The environment needs to be unpressured and quiet. Care workers need to provide the opportunity for the client to talk about how they are feeling. If the client cannot communicate well, the carer has to try and validate their feelings and acknowledge their depression. Activity should be encouraged as a form of distraction, but also as an antidote in itself, to depressive thoughts and feelings. Engaging in pleasurable activity is a form of treatment in its own right. Depression saps the energy and inclination to engage with what we previously found pleasurable. Engaging a client in activity can help enormously in breaking this pattern.

Achievement in activities allows us to give praise and positive reinforcement as to the client's abilities.

We, as carers, also need to be able to speak out and advocate on behalf of our clients – even more so if they are depressed. It is bad enough having a dementia, but having a treatable depression on top of this, and not getting treatment which can help, is an unforgivable state of affairs (see a checklist of indicators of depression in older people on p.207).

Health and Social Care National Occupational Standards

This chapter relates to many of the induction and foundation standards but in particular to the following level standards:

Level 2 core units

HSC24b Treat people with respect and dignity.
HSC226 a, b + c Support individuals who are distressed.

Level 3 optional units

HSC331 a, b + c Support individuals to develop and maintain social networks and relationships.
HSC396 b +c Work with people to review the effectiveness of their coping strategies and develop alternatives.

Level 4 optional units

HSC418a Obtain information about individuals' mental health needs.

Mental Health Standards

A4.1, 4.2 Promote effective communication and relationships.
A6.1, 6.2, 6.3 Promote effective communication where there are communication differences.
A5.1, 5.2 Promote effective communication and relationships with people who are troubled or distressed.
J2.1, 2.2 Support individuals when they are distressed.

Care Homes for Older People: National Minimum Standards

8.1 Promote and maintain service users' health and ensure access to health care services to meet assessed needs.
8.7 The service user's psychological health is monitored regularly and preventative and restorative care provided.
10.5 Treat people with respect at all times.
12.3 Service users are given the opportunity to pursue leisure activities in keeping with their interests. Particular consideration is given to people with dementia.

Exercise 31.1

A CHECKLIST OF INDICATORS OF DEPRESSION IN OLDER PEOPLE

- Low mood.

- Thoughts of death and suicidal ideas.

- Feelings of hopelessness and worthlessness.

- Low self-esteem.

- Reduced appetite confirmed by weight loss (but on rare occasions there is weight gain via comfort eating).

- Sleep disturbance, typically waking early in the morning or having difficulty getting to sleep.

- Agitation and anxiety, typically restlessness and pacing to and fro.

- Loss of interest in, for example, hobbies and activities of daily living.

- Reduced personal hygiene and appearance.

- Withdrawal, isolation and reduced communication.

- Poor concentration.

- Poor memory.

- Physical slowing down, slowness of speech and movement.

- Loss of energy, fatigue.

- Hypochondria is a common feature of depression in older people: they will complain of many physical ills.

Remember:

- These signs may be hard to detect in clients with dementia.

- Many of these signs are common features of life generally. It is when several of them occur together and persist over time that depression may be present.

Chapter 32

Drugs and Dementia

Key messages

- Medication to control behaviour is always a last resort. There are many other tactics that can be tried first.
- Medication can increase confusion and physical vulnerability.
- Medication issues should be discussed by as wide a group as possible and always include family and close friends.

There are several aspects of the use of medication in dementia care which are worthy of examination. The new acetylcholinesterase inhibitor drugs which are said to combat dementia and the use of medication to control behaviour are both important issues. The use of covert medication and the role of complementary therapy also need some discussion.

Anti-dementia drugs

The popular term 'anti-dementia drugs' masks the truth that there is still no cure for dementia. What these drugs can do though is to slow down the effects of the dementia upon the person by diminishing the symptoms for a period of time. The drugs maintain the person's level of functioning but the disease is still progressing.

How do they work?

Drugs have both brand and chemical names and the commonest of these drugs are Aricept (donepezil hydrochloride), Exelon (rivastigmine) and Reminyl (galantamine).

These drugs are called 'acetylcholinesterase inhibitors'. In Alzheimer's there is a reduction in the amount of acetylcholine in the brain and this chemical helps nerve cells to communicate with each other. Acetylcholine is normally broken down by an enzyme called 'acetylcholinesterase'. Exelon, Aricept and Reminyl work by inhibiting this enzyme and thus increasing the amount of acetylcholine in the brain. The result is an improvement in symptoms or a halting of further decline.

Another drug, Exiba (memantine), acts in a different way to produce similar effects.

Who will they work for?

Much more research needs to be carried out upon the effectiveness of these drugs, but at present Aricept, Exelon and Reminyl are used in mild to moderate dementia. Exiba is said to be effective in moderate to severe dementia. The drugs, however, do not work for everyone and their effects are only temporary. A temporary reduction in symptoms and some respite from the progression of the disease is, however, no small thing.

Benefits

The benefit of these drugs is the slowing down of the progression of the dementia. The evidence from the Alzheimer's Society's own research (Alzheimer's Society 2000) indicates that they can give a substantial improvement not in cognitive performance but in mood and an enthusiasm for life. They report that the new drugs also considerably reduce anxiety and stress and restore sufferers' confidence. The research also found that social interaction and communication skills improved. This increased confidence brings about a significant improvement in performance of activities of daily living.

Decline

As the disease progresses less and less acetylcholine is produced for the drugs to work on with a subsequent lack of benefit. This is why the drugs are only effective in the early stages of dementia. Eventually the drug has no effect and once this stage has been reached the condition of the sufferer will, over a month or so, reach the stage they would have been at had they not taken the drug. So the disease has progressed but the symptoms have been kept at bay (see Figure 32.1). The sufferer has temporarily gained a period of improved quality of life.

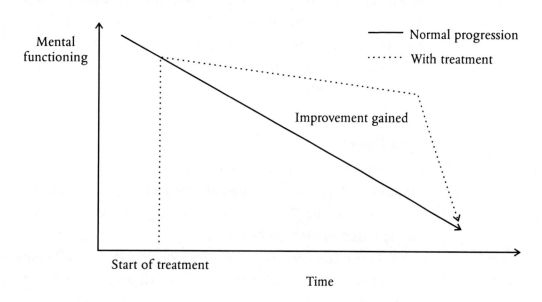

Figure 32.1 Reduced decline in functioning with anti-dementia drugs

It can be seen from Figure 32.1 that there is a considerable area of improved quality of life which can result from treatment. This can mean an enormous amount to both sufferers and family carers.

Medication and 'problem' behaviour

See Exercise 32.2, p.216.

Medication for disturbed behaviour

Medication is all too often a first response to 'problem' behaviours which carers find difficult to manage or tolerate. Aggressive or antisocial behaviour is often thus tranquillised before any attempt is made to understand it or work with the sufferer displaying such behaviours. The use of anti-psychotic medication will subdue both the behaviour and the person, and continued use will render the person apathetic, withdrawn and lifeless as well as subjecting them to unpleasant side effects. Older people are also often more prone to the side effects of constipation, tremors, excessive salivation and sedation. When you think about it, it seems quite unreasonable to give a medication which 'fogs' the brain to a person whose brain is already 'fogged' by their dementia.

The use of medication is often merely a lazy way of coping. It is an easy way of coping with difficult (for us) behaviours. It does away with awkward situations and allows things to become more manageable. However getting rid of the 'problem' often also gets rid of the person. When faced with an awkward behaviour we should try to look for a range of possible reasons for it. Having done this it is often easier to see a range of possible solutions. These might work or you might have to think of other ways, but in general you will usually hit upon a solution. The use of medication in such circumstances should always be the last option. Chapter 13 on problem solving and the chapters on different so-called 'problem behaviours' will help you to explore the range of possible reasons and solutions. Commonly, difficult behaviour arises out of boredom and a lack of stimulation and interaction. By using medication we are often just treating the symptom not the cause.

Major tranquillisers

The drugs used for agitation and aggression are usually anti-psychotics (major tranquillisers) used for treating delusions and hallucinations in illnesses such as schizophrenia. They have a rapid and strong sedative effect and this is the reason they are used to manage behaviour.

Where medication is used it is important that care staff monitor its effectiveness and are aware of what the possible side effects are. Carers are in the best position to monitor these things as they spend most time with the client. It is also important that carers ensure that the medication is reviewed on a regular basis.

Side effects of major tranquillisers

Side effects include over-sedation, low blood pressure leading to falls especially on standing up, tremor and stiffness of the limbs, dry mouth, blurred vision and constipation.

Anti-anxiety drugs

Anti-anxiety drugs are called 'benzodiazepines', common ones being Valium and Lorazepam. They are useful for acute anxiety or panic states. They bring quick relief via sedation and thus it is important to guard against any resulting unsteadiness which can lead to falls. They are also extremely addictive and should not be given for longer than two weeks. There is a trade-off between reducing the agitation and distress to the sufferer but enhancing confusion and unsteadiness.

Antidepressants

If you think about it, it is easy to see why many people suffering confusion and dementia become depressed. In the early stages an awareness of your failing mind is likely to cause depression. Wattis and Curran (2001) suggest that those with early dementia are twice as likely to be depressed as the general population. Later on, as the disease progresses further, not being able to make sense of the world around you or communicate effectively with it must be very frustrating and frightening. Any insight will increase these feelings and can lead to severe depression. In such cases antidepressant medication might be needed. Far more important though is good care. Understanding how the sufferer is feeling and communicating that to them, giving them time, contact and displaying concern will be invaluable in helping to lift depression. By showing you care and that you value the person you are helping them to feel less isolated in their depression.

Where the depression persists and is not amenable to other interventions, antidepressants can be very useful. It is important that they are taken regularly and for up to six months to prevent a relapse. They can take up to three weeks or more to have an effect. It is also important that the sufferer is monitored for side effects.

There are various types of antidepressants. Older drugs called 'tricyclic antidepressants' are very toxic in overdose and have quite severe side effects such as drowsiness, dry mouth, blurred vision, dizziness and difficulty urinating. There are also some more recent antidepressants called 'SSRIs' which, not having such bad side effects, may be more suitable.

Covert medication

There are many difficult questions which need answering in relation to the use of covert medication. Exercise 32.2, p.216 attempts to address the major ones.

Good practice

Where the client is unable to give consent it is good practice to consult with the nearest relative and others concerned with their care.

The decision to use covert medication should be taken at a team meeting or case conference where as many opinions as possible are taken into account. The team should be sure that the action is in the patient's best interests and not solely to ease management of difficult behaviour. This is a safeguard against abuse.

An attempt should be made to explain to the person afterwards that they were given medication to calm them down as it was felt to be in their best interests.

All incidents of covert use of medication should be recorded in the client's notes. The record should document the reason for its use including both staff and skill shortages.

Treat each case differently and each decision afresh. Often abuse arises because one incident of covert medication was justified and it then becomes standard practice.

Complementary therapy

Whilst the evidence for effectiveness of complementary therapies might be questioned by some, it is clear that it has a valuable role to play in enhancing the quality of life of dementia sufferers. Massage, aromatherapy, relaxation therapy, acupuncture and herbal medicine are just a few of the many alternative approaches to health care which can be used in conjunction with the more conventional treatments.

Much of the value of complementary medicine in dementia care is in inducing a calm and relaxed state. It is suggested that lavender oil, for example, has an effect in reducing agitation. Massage, relaxation and aromatherapy are all well within the capabilities of most care staff (see Exercise 32.3, p.217). The increased level of interaction and physical contact that comes from using such therapies will also be of enormous benefit.

The politics of medication

It is evident that in many long-stay institutions there is a serious staffing shortage. Because of this the temptation arises to use sedative drugs to make life easier for the staff. This is clearly wrong but also probably quite widespread. The only real solution is to provide adequate numbers of well trained staff.

This is not some glib accusation but an acknowledgement of the reality for dementia sufferers in many nursing and residential homes.

Positive drug use

Medication should only be used as a last resort and for good reason for if it is not then it is merely a form of chemical restraint and thus abuse. It is also worth remembering that anything that sedates can quite easily add to a person's confusion.

There may of course be times when a sufferer becomes very distressed and cannot be comforted no matter what you try. When this is the case and the distress it causes persists then it is justifiable to use medication to alleviate the distress. Such ethical use is in the interest of the client. The danger is that this becomes a routine response to behaviour that we find hard to tolerate.

Health and Social Care National Occupational Standards

This chapter relates to many of the induction and foundation standards but in particular to the following level standards:

Level 3 optional units

HSC375 a + b Administer medication to individuals.

HSC3119 a, b + c Promote the values and principles underpinning best practice. Challenge poor practice and be open to challenge by others.

Level 4 optional units

HSC414a Work with individuals to assess their needs and preferences.

Care Homes for Older People: National Minimum Standards

9.1 to 9.11 All refer to medication, largely with respect to storage and handling, but 9.10 requires that medication is reviewed on a regular basis.

Further reading and references

Alzheimer's Society (2000) *Appraisal of the Drugs for Alzheimer's Disease: Submission to the National Institute for Clinical Excellence.* London: Alzheimer's Society.

This is a report by the Alzheimer's Society to the National Institute for Clinical Excellence in relation to the new anticholinesterase drug treatments. In its introduction it gives the powerful statement that, were it not for these drugs, it would not have been possible to include the views of sufferers. They argue that we are learning much as a result of the new drugs enabling people with Alzheimer's to talk about their experience. The report was compiled from questionnaire responses of people with Alzheimer's and their carers. The report is worth reading for the insight it gives into what it must be like to both suffer and care. It expresses the views of both in a way that conventional research often ignores and in doing so offers us a remarkable insight. The report emphasises the value of the additional years of quality of life the new drugs give. Because of the temporary nature of the improvement it is described as 'borrowed time'. The report concluded that 73 per cent of their respondents felt that the new drugs worked.

Alzheimer's Society (2004) *Dementia: Drugs Used to Relieve Behavioural Symptoms.* Information sheet available from www.alzheimers.org.uk

Alzheimer's Society (2003) *Drug Treatments for Alzheimer's.* Fact sheet available from www.alzheimers.org.uk

Wattis, J. and Curran, S. (eds) (2001) *Practical Psychiatry of Old Age.* Third edition. Oxford: Radcliffe Medical Press.

This is a classic and well-written text book which gives a clear introduction to the use of drugs in dementia. The book reiterates the fact that medication should be the last resort as there are often other obvious causal reasons for distress, such as environmental discomfort and lack of stimulation.

AVOIDING SEDATION

Brian had always been a bit of a leader; he liked to take control in his life. He had many proud achievements. He was always on the go, always doing something related to his many hobbies and interests. His career as a head teacher meant that he was used to being in control and respected.

After his dementia worsened Brian's wife had to take the decision to find him a specialist nursing home so that she could have a break. She could no longer cope with his wandering and 'interfering' and he had become doubly incontinent and somewhat argumentative. She still loved him dearly and wanted to continue caring for him but badly needed a break. She was in tears as she left Brian at the home for a week's respite and promised him she would visit during the week. After two days had gone by she could bear it no longer, she was worried he would be missing her and scared of the strange surroundings.

She rang the home to say she would visit and was reassured that he was OK by the nurse telling her he was settled. When she arrived and saw Brian she was horrified to find him slumped in an armchair, drooling saliva from his mouth. He could barely sit up and couldn't speak. He was clearly over-sedated and could not walk. She thought he'd had a heart attack or stroke and when she asked what had happened, she was told that he had become agitated when she'd left, he tried to get out and when he was redirected the agitation turned into aggression. The other residents were frightened and staff reluctant to tolerate him. The duty doctor was called and he prescribed him an anti-psychotic drug to calm him down. It worked well and he had been given it several more times to keep him calm.

- What possible reasons might there be to explain Brian's agitation?

- How might it have been managed without medication?

- If all the strategies you can think of did not work, what else could be done to help the situation?

Exercise 32.2

COVERT MEDICATION ISSUES

This is David's second time on respite at the care home and he is clearly not happy at being there. Despite the best efforts of the staff he cannot be calmed down and is beginning to get aggressive. The GP has prescribed him a tranquilliser to help calm him down but he refuses to take it and has hit out at a nurse who tried to persuade him to do so. David is now banging on doors and windows becoming quite agitated and clearly distressed. The staff nurse approaches him calmly and manages to get him to sit down and accept a cup of tea. He drinks the tea quickly and immediately becomes agitated again. However, within fifteen minutes he has sat down and become quiet. It is not long before he is fast asleep in the chair.

The nurse has put his liquid tranquilliser in his tea. This act raises several ethical issues to do with the use of covert medication.

There are no easy answers here, but we can identify both good practices and unethical approaches which will better inform our decisions in every case.

- David had not consented to take the medication so was it morally right to trick him into taking it?

- What are the arguments *for* the use of such tactics?

- What are the arguments against?

- Was the action in the best interests of the patient to preserve their well-being?

- If we can see someone is clearly distressed and we have the power to help them, is it not morally correct to give the medication?

- Does the risk of falls outweigh the calming effect of the medication?

- To do anything against the wishes of the person is to disregard their human rights. We are giving the person the message that they are not important or worthy of rights. Do we not distance ourselves further from the person and reduce the chances of them ever believing or trusting us again?

- Covert medication is often used simply because units are understaffed and cannot therefore deal with the behaviour. Is this justified?

Exercise 32.3

ALTERNATIVES

- Think about your clients and whether there is the opportunity to introduce some forms of complementary therapy such as a combined relaxation and aromatherapy session, or a massage routine.

- Draw up a list of clients and think about how they might be helped by alternative therapies.

- Remember it may be possible to enlist the help of local practitioners to teach you the basics so that you can provide the therapy yourselves.

Exercise 32.4

TREATMENT OR ABUSE?

With a group of colleagues try and discuss these views and consider the following questions:

- In the private sector does the need to balance the books take priority over adequate staffing levels?

- Are clients under-stimulated and is this a cause of distress?

- Does your establishment use drugs to manage situations because you have not got the staff or the time to deal with the problem?

- If this is the case in a nursing home what could the staff do about it?

Chapter 33

Ethical Considerations

Key messages

- A diagnosis of dementia does not take away your capacity to consent or refuse.
- Even those with advanced dementia are capable of making some choices.

Ethics does not give us answers, it merely gives us different ways of looking at things. This, in itself, however, is immensely helpful. When a difficult decision has to be made, it is wise to gather as many opinions as possible. Doing so eliminates some of the risk of individual bias and spreading the responsibility helps to eradicate extremes, so that what is left is the consensus view. A decision taken in this way is nearly always safer and more rational than one taken in isolation. Sharing thoughts on difficult ethical dilemmas will likewise help to achieve a more morally sound outcome. This is not to say that we should be blind to extremes or that we should always strive for the middle way. We still need to be open to radical solutions and to tearing up the rule book in order to achieve a morally sound outcome.

Restraint

Restraint is an important issue as often the distinction between care and abuse is blurred.

Autonomy

Literally, 'autonomy' means 'self-rule'. Can the person direct their own actions? The uninformed conclusion is that people with a dementia cannot do this, but it is not quite that simple. People in the early stages of dementia clearly are fully autonomous. In the latter stages too people with a dementia clearly do direct their own actions within that dementia: they have autonomy within the dementia. Seldom is wandering or any other behaviour purposeless. It nearly always has meaning to the client, even when we cannot understand it. The person with dementia still has thoughts and feelings which direct their behaviour. Even in memory loss where the client strives to recall their past and who they are, this does not strip them of their autonomy. When communication ability is lost clients may take the autonomous decision to withdraw from the world to protect themselves from further anxiety-provoking experiences.

Autonomy is also bound up with the freedom to make choices and in many ways institutional care, not the dementia, strips away this freedom. Ethically we should be protecting a person's autonomy, not eroding it. We should be encouraging the range of choices open to clients.

Competence

Competence is similar to autonomy, the question being: is the person in control of their situation? The progress of a dementia and the cognitive decline which that brings clearly erodes such competence. There quite clearly comes a point where the client cannot make decisions about their own life, and we have to accept this, but it does not mean that they are totally incapable of making choices, or devoid of any individuality or personality. We might have to act on their behalf in the light of their assumed wishes and we can attempt to do so, but only if we know the client well. We can do not what we think is best for them, but what we think they would have wanted given their unique history, beliefs and views. The need to consult with family, relatives and friends is obvious in order to gain an idea of their wishes. The carer must consult those who know the client in regard to important decisions and choices.

Advanced directives

These are statements of how the client wants to be treated and should be drawn up in the early stages of a dementia. The client highlights what their preferences and wishes are should they not be able to make decisions for themselves. They are invaluable in allowing us to make decisions in keeping with the individual's wishes once they have lost the capacity to inform us. They can cover anything from what the person likes to wear to what medical treatment they prefer to whether they want to be kept alive artificially. These decisions when at the life-and-death end of the spectrum are very difficult – there is seldom a clear-cut, easily decided way forward – but an advanced directive can at least inform us of what the client's wishes would be.

The difficulty arises in judging when a person becomes incompetent because of their dementia and at what point should we rely on their advanced directive rather than their currently expressed wishes. The obvious answer is that if the client can still express a wish then it is too early to look at the advanced directive. The picture is clouded by the fact that a person might change because of the dementia: their experience of dementia might have made them change in what they want, from the time when they wrote the directive.

Personhood

There is always a person inside the dementia. This should be a guiding principle behind all our care. The person is always there and the drive to foster this uniqueness and personality, to achieve good, person centred care, must be at the heart of all care work. Not to do this is to relegate the person to a mere collection of troublesome behaviours. When this becomes the case clients are often subjected to the forms of bad care Kitwood (1997) describes as 'malignant social psychology'. They are no longer regarded as real people. Philosophers can play with words and semantics and argue that where there is no rationality, no ability to make decisions, no ability to self-direct, no autonomy, then there is no personhood. However, even in the deepest dementia there remains the ability to smile, to have feelings and emotions, to be happy or sad, and because of this personhood remains intact throughout. Such a person deserves dignity and respect and one can argue that the lack of person centred care and denial of individuality are a form of abuse.

Truth telling

The question to be asked when it comes to being truthful or not with clients is: 'In whose interests am I doing this?' Often lies are used in dementia care for the convenience of the staff. It is far easier to say, 'Come on, it'll be all right, they'll be back in five minutes, let's have a cup of tea' to a client who is upset at a visitor leaving. It is done in a well-meaning way, to minimise distress, but it ignores and invalidates the client's feelings and dismisses them as unimportant. We need to acknowledge distress and let clients know we recognise their distress – then comfort them with the offer of a drink. Far too many carers and nurses shy away from difficult emotional situations, but doing so in dementia care invalidates that person's very existence. Not telling the truth will also quickly erode any trust the client had in you. At any stage of dementia honesty and truth telling are essential if we are not to undermine the client's confidence and trust. If they cannot trust us who can they turn to? They will become completely alone in a world where even those who are supposed to care for them will not tell them the truth.

Consent

In order not to override the person's autonomy, even in cases where it is assumed they have none left, we should always seek consent. It is polite to ask a person's permission, for example, before entering their room. This is a central part of person centred care. Not to seek simple permission is tantamount to saying that the client does not matter, they are not worth bothering with, not worthy of respect. So, even where the client cannot give consent, it should still be sought.

> **Discussion point**
>
> - Does cognitive testing as part of assessments do more harm that good?
>
> - By repeatedly putting clients through such tests to record assumed decline in ability, are we not just giving them frequent traumatic reminders of what cognitive failings they have?
>
> - By mixing clients with relatively early dementia with other clients with late-stage dementia on assessment wards, are we not guilty of cruelty?

Health and Social Care National Occupational Standards

This chapter relates to many of the induction and foundation standards but in particular to the following level standards:

Level 2 core units

HSC24 a, b +c Ensure your actions support the care, protection and well being of individuals.

Level 2 optional units

HSC234 a, b + c Ensure your actions support the equality, diversity, rights and responsibilities of individuals.

Level 3 optional units

HSC3111 a, b + c Promote the equality, diversity, rights and responsibilities of individuals.

HSC3119c Challenge poor practice and be open to challenge by others.

Level 4 optional units

HSC410c Advocate for, and with, individuals and carers.

HSC414a Work with individuals to assess their needs and preferences.

Mental Health Standards

A3.1, 3.2, 3.3 Promote the values and principles underpinning best practice.

Care Homes for Older People: National Minimum Standards

14.1 The home maximises the service user's capacity to exercise personal autonomy and choice.

Further reading and references

Cameron, S. (1998) 'Whose life is it anyway?' In P. Barker and B. Davidson (eds) *Psychiatric Nursing: Ethical Strife*. London: Arnold.

Hunter, S. (ed.) (1997) *Dementia: Challenges and New Directions*. London: Jessica Kingsley Publishers.

Kitwood, T. (1997) *Dementia Reconsidered. The Person Comes First*. Buckingham: Open University Press.

Jacques, A. (1997) 'Ethical dilemmas in care and research for people with dementia.' In S. Hunter (ed.) *Dementia: Challenges and New Directions*. London: Jessica Kingsley Publishers.

Exercise 33.1
IS IT ETHICALLY ALL RIGHT TO...

- lock the doors?

- sit a person in a chair they cannot get out of?

- medicate difficult behaviour rather than try to understand it and work with it?

- get everybody up at the same time?

- provide no activity or stimulation?

For each of these scenarios list the possible reasons as to why they occur.

Try and come up with more ethically acceptable and practical solutions for each of the scenarios.

Then ask what you as a team can do about similar scenarios in your care environment.

What other aspects of practice might be considered ethically dubious?

Generate a list and then examine ways of avoiding such practices.

Chapter 34

Early Onset Dementia

Key messages

- Early onset dementia is more common than the statistics show, as it is often not diagnosed until much later.
- Sufferers have particular and special needs, yet there are few specialist or age-appropriate services available.

A dementia afflicting people earlier in life is tragic. Many areas of the country have no specialist social service or NHS facilities for helping people with early onset dementia. The care a sufferer receives is still something of a lottery depending upon where you live and what sort of priority the local authorities place upon it. Often people are inappropriately placed in care homes for people much older than themselves simply because no other care facility has the expertise in dealing with dementia. The Alzheimer's Society estimate that in 2001 there were roughly 18,500 people under 65 years old with dementia. The majority of these had Alzheimer's disease, but there is also a greater prevalence of the rarer dementias such as multiple sclerosis and Parkinson's disease. Other forms of dementia occurring at younger ages are Creutzfeldt–Jakobs disease, Down's Syndrome dementia, Pick's disease, frontal lobe damage and AIDS dementia.

Caring for someone with early onset dementia in a care setting geared to older people can be fraught with difficulty. The levels of frustration in sufferers in the early stages, whilst insight remains, are huge. It is difficult for a sufferer to accept such a loss of skills at so early an age. By the time the person has entered care they will have had to deal with:

- coping with personal life issues such as relationships, sex, reduced ability with personal care and reduced capacity to perform activities of daily living

- dealing with the effects upon their often young, dependent children

- dealing with issues related to work, such as how or whether to continue with it

- eventually having to cease work. This will entail issues such as loss of role, self-esteem, money and activity

- dealing with the effects of loss of income, which have repercussions for pension rights and mortgage payments, all of which will cause anxiety

- having to seek legal advice about wills and power of attorney

- having to stop driving

- probably having been severely depressed.

The task for care workers is to ensure that the client receives age appropriate care. Care workers will have the skills for caring for the dementia and its effects upon the client, but these need to be applied and practised in the context of a younger person. A person centred care approach remains appropriate here but care must be taken that the sufferer is not drawn into a culture and age which is inappropriate to them. Enlisting the help of relatives and friends, with care plans drawn up in consultation with these close personal contacts, will help to ensure this does not happen.

Chapter 35

Supporting and Including Relatives and Friends

Key message

Family and friends are key components of care.

It is easy to forget the needs of relatives and friends of clients who visit them. Carers can be too busy and focused upon the needs of the client to recognise the needs of visitors. Yet this is a very important aspect of care work. Visitors have very real needs for support, understanding and involvement and providing such will also bring benefits for the clients.

The decision to place a loved one in care is never an easy one. Often it is a last resort and a time of extreme trauma and sadness. Relatives have not abandoned the person, they are quite simply often mentally and physically exhausted and no longer capable of caring at home without the resources available in a care home. There will be a deep sense of loss and grief which can be made worse by underlying guilt at having let the person down or feelings of having failed the person they love. There will also be some loneliness and anxiety that no one will be able to provide care in the way they did. There may also be feelings of relief that someone else is taking over, especially if it has been difficult for them to cope.

It is likely that there will be a mixture of all of these and the relative often needs to talk about their feelings with a sympathetic listener.

Most carers will be capable of listening and understanding the real difficulties the relative has faced by virtue of their own experience of working with clients suffering from dementia. Such an understanding allows the carer to provide empathy rather than just sympathy. You should make time for listening to relatives, especially around the time of admission as this is an important form of support. You can try to dispel their feelings of guilt by emphasising that they have made the right decision. To a large extent guilt is eroded by making the relative aware that their loved one is still loved, being well cared for and treated as an individual. The most important way of putting their mind at rest is the attitude of the care staff towards the clients. They need to see that you care beyond the physical and daily routine care work. They need to perceive love and that you are interested in the whole person. Sometimes relatives cannot deal with the guilt immediately and it can drive them to complain about the care their loved one is receiving. This is another opportunity, not to get defensive, but to listen to them and allow them to talk about their experiences and feelings. A good care worker will acknowledge such complaints as an expression of guilt and loss. By allowing this expression, giving time and listening, the care worker can relieve the feelings the relative is experiencing.

Hidden victims

Relatives and home carers have often coped admirably with severe problems, limited resources and little acknowledgement. Caring for a person with dementia in a care-home setting is much easier than coping with it in the outside world. The general public and authorities can be very unsympathetic. Caring at home has been described by Mace and Rabins (1985) as the 36-hour day. They described the 'burden' of caring as consisting of dealing with aggression, incontinence, changed personality, wandering, withdrawal, non-communication, repetition, sleep disturbance, uncertainty, loss of partner, deteriorating habits, loss of social life and isolation, to name just a few. All of which adds up to a very tiring and stressful existence. Many carers do not receive financial help and have given up work. There is often little community support and many do not receive any practical help or respite of any kind. If it were not for the efforts of the Alzheimer's Society many would receive no help at all.

Discussion point

Whilst on placement at a nursing home for clients with dementia, two student nurses were asked to go into the local town and find out what support and services were out there for people with dementia and those looking after them. They returned at the end of the day very frustrated and saddened.

- What support is there for dementia sufferers and the people looking after them in your local area?

- If you are not sure repeat the students' exercise.

Involvement

Care homes are busy places and should embrace the willingness of relatives and friends to get involved. The involvement of relatives might need to be instigated by the care staff as many will feel it is not their place or that they are interfering. Yet around the time of admission it is often very therapeutic for the relative to feel that they can still be involved and can still provide care for their spouse. This will help to dispel thoughts that they have abandoned their loved one. It will also help combat the sudden loss of role and purpose they had when caring at home.

It is important to remember that the relationship stays the same. The client is still their husband, wife, son, daughter or best friend etc. They are just living in the care home so, where relatives want to, carers should try to encourage as near normal a relationship as possible. Providing the opportunity for intimacy and privacy is especially important here. Equally important is the relative's continued opportunity to be involved in the normal everyday aspects of life for their loved one such as dressing, shopping, dining, activity, personal care etc.

Relatives are the experts in caring for our clients and we should make them feel such by constantly seeking their guidance and involvement. They need to feel that they are the client's key worker and in charge of their care: just because they are living within your care home does not mean that the relative has abandoned responsibility for their care. Only by such involvement will we be able to get to know the client better and so tailor our care more to their unique needs. We should use and be directed by the relatives.

Discussion point

- In what ways can you encourage a relative to become more involved in the care of the client?
- What aspects of your routine get in the way of relative involvement?
- How can you overcome these?

Other important aspects of relatives involvement are:

- putting together a life story and scrapbook of the client's life
- involving them in care planning and reviews
- involving them in the organisation and daily life of the care home
- involving them in fundraising
- starting a relatives' group
- bringing in personal possessions
- decorating the client's room
- running parties.

There will, of course, be relatives who want no further involvement and this should be respected. It can be quite natural for people to feel this way, especially if it has been a very long struggle to cope. Community services to support carers of people with dementia are often pitiful, reflecting perhaps a low priority given to dementia by society. However, it is prudent to offer an ear and listen to their story and respect their wish for a break. It is also prudent to leave the door open for future involvement by occasionally testing the waters and offering the opportunity to help.

Death

When a death nears relatives might either shy away or want to have more involvement. You will need to support both options. Many will be glad to be involved up until the moment death occurs and might even want to help with last offices. When a death occurs, the relative who has visited often and become part of the routine of the home will feel a great sense of loss for their loved one. Having become a large part of their lives it might be you who they turn to for consolation and help to deal with their grief. It is important that you are available for the relative and make time to listen and encourage them to talk about their sorrow and reminisce about the good times too. This all helps people to come to terms with the loss. However, it might be that the relative is also sad at losing their involvement and role within the home and if this is so you should facilitate their continued involvement.

Health and Social Care National Occupational Standards

This chapter relates to many of the induction and foundation standards but in particular to the following level standards:

Level 2 optional units

HSC226c Support individuals through periods of stress and distress.
HSC227a Contribute to working in collaboration with carers to identify their needs and preferences.
HSC245 a, b + c Receive and monitor visitors.

Level 3 optional units

HSC387 a, b + c Work in collaboration with carers in the caring role.
HSC388 a, b + c Relate to families and carers.

Mental Health Standards

C2.1, 2.2, 2.3, 2.4 Develop, implement and review programmes of support for carers and families.
C6.1 Promote the contribution of families, carers and others to supporting individuals with mental health needs.

Care Homes for Older People: National Minimum Standards

10.1 and 10.2 These relate to issues of dignity and maintaining contact with relatives and friends.

13.1 to 13.6 These relate to maintaining contact with families and the wider community.

Further reading and references

Benson, S. (ed.) (1992) *The Care Assistants Guide to Working with People with Dementia*. London: Journal of Dementia Care.

Mace, L., Rabins, P., Castleton, C., Cloke, C. and McEwan, E. (1985) *The 36 Hour Day: Caring at Home for Confused Elderly People*. Sevenoaks: Hodder and Stoughton/Age Concern.

Chapter 36

Supporting Each Other

Key message
Happy and valued staff usually means happy clients.

> **Discussion point**
>
> - List those aspects of care work which demoralise staff: think about the care home you work in and your own experiences.
>
> - What causes each of these?
>
> - For each example you find brain storm ways of improving the situation.
>
> - If you were the manager of your home, what would you do to improve staff morale?

Caring for people suffering with dementia is one of the most demanding of caring tasks. It requires great skill, patience, love, mental and physical stamina, practicality and humour, to name just a few qualities. Such a mixture of skills is rare and yet is greatly undervalued and under-rewarded. The great majority of those who work most closely with clients with dementia, those who do most of the day-to-day caring, are care assistants. For many, there are greater financial rewards to be had working in the local supermarket. This is a sad indictment which reflects the low priority we as a society place on the continuing care of older people with dementia and older people generally.

Given this situation it is essential that care staff are well supported if they are not to burn out and become disillusioned. A large part of this means supporting each other. The rest is support from trained staff, managers and training programmes.

Recognising staff skills

A useful starting point for managers is in recognising the experience and skills of care staff and utilising these in a positive and rewarding way for both clients and staff. A gift for gardening, for example, can be put to good use to offer clients an activity and is an opportunity to offer praise to the colleague concerned.

Shared teaching

Apart from formal training programmes, there are training sessions which can be organised which centre upon using the expertise of the care staff. Case discussions and problem-solving workshops are especially useful here.

Variety

It is important to give care staff responsibilities beyond their normal caring role. Such responsibilities might be certain management functions and activity functions such as organising events, fundraising and report writing.

Staff meetings

Managers need to ensure that these are regular and are not just of an administrative and problem discussion nature. There need to be staff meetings of a clinical nature where the goal of quality of life of the clients is the central theme for discussion. But also staff meetings are a way of finding out the concerns of the care staff and of asking what their support needs are. Managers should not assume that they know this; they must ask regularly.

Case conferences

Care staff should be given associate key worker responsibility for named clients and should be involved in writing up case notes and reports. They should also be involved in case conferences and their opinions actively sought.

Time

There is an assumption that once a week you can all meet to discuss the questions raised in this book or have other training inputs. If this is not the case, ask the manager to arrange it so that such sessions can happen and ask them to facilitate them or to ask one of the trained nurses if they are willing to do so. Point out the training and supportive functions that such a weekly session would bring.

Students

Does your home provide placements for student nurses and other students? If not discuss this possibility with your manager. Student nurses will need a qualified member of staff to mentor them and will need care assistants to 'buddy' them. Care assistants make a huge contribution to nurse education in this way by passing on their skills and acting as role models in dealing with difficult situations. They are also invaluable in passing on their many practical skills. This is another opportunity for care assistants to be involved in training by providing short sessions for the student nurses. Such responsibility raises the status of the care assistant and managers should note that the resulting increased self-esteem will have positive returns for client care.

Health and Social Care National Occupational Standards

This chapter relates to many of the induction and foundation standards but in particular to the following level standards:

Level 2 core units

HSC23 a + b Develop your knowledge and practice.

Level 2 optional units

HSC228 a, b + c Contribute to effective group care.
HSC241 a + b Contribute to the effectiveness of teams.

Level 3 core units

HSC33 a + b Reflect and develop your practice.

Level 3 optional units

HSC3100 a, b + c Participate in interdisciplinary team working to support individuals.
HSC3110 a, b + c Support colleagues to relate to individuals.
HSC3119 a, b + c Promote the values and principles underpinning best practice.
HSC3120b Give staff members support in the workplace and feedback on their performance.
HSC3121 a, b + c Contribute to promoting the effectiveness of teams.

Level 4 core units

HSC43 a + b Take responsibility for the continuing professional development of self and others.

Mental Health Standards

A1.1, 1.2 Develop your own knowledge and practice.
A2.1, 2.2 Reflect upon and develop practice using supervision and support.
A3.1, 3.2, 3.3 Promote the values and principles underpinning best practice.

Care Homes for Older People: National Minimum Standards

30.1 to 30.4 These relate to staff training, including induction and beyond, to ensure that all staff are competent.
36.1 to 36.5 These relate to ensuring that all staff receive appropriate supervision covering all aspects of practice.

Further reading and references

Norman, I. (1997) 'Supporting paid carers.' In I. Norman and S. Redfern (eds) *Mental Health Care for Elderly People.* Edinburgh: Churchill Livingstone.

✓

Exercise 36.1

PERSONAL TRAINING NEEDS

In a group think of all the training sessions you would like to have. Then invite your manager to the meeting and discuss the possibilities of your list. Think about those outside speakers who might come in and give a half-hour talk followed by a half-hour question-and-answer session.

Exercise 36.2

GIVING

- As a staff group of care assistants imagine that you have a school leaver starting. What half-hour training sessions could *you* give?

- List these down and take one each week and discuss what would need to go into the training session.

- Prepare flip charts of bullet points for each session.

Postscript

If you are feeling disheartened by the fact that the work you do is hard, under-valued, under-rewarded and mentally and physically shattering, then you would be right. But be reminded also that to the people you look after, you are their link to life, their support and their advocate. To some you will be their only friend, the only one they recognise and trust. To the client with dementia you may well be their only link to reality, to a world they find increasingly difficult to engage with and understand. You may be the one thing that gives them hope and keeps away the fear that losing your mind must surely bring. Beyond this you must strive to validate their world. They are at your mercy, no one else will understand. The reason you can help them is because you have taken the time to get to know them as individuals and treated them as such. You will recognise just what a huge privilege this is, as few get as close to the clients as you. You will in-variably say that you do it because you care, you like people and you don't seek financial reward.

The world owes the care assistant a huge debt of gratitude. However, there comes a time when such devotion should be rewarded, and when the skills, knowledge and attitudes you have should be rewarded and taken further.

Your knowledge and skills will see you through NVQ courses and gain you nationally recognised qualifications.

Consideration should also be given to undertaking nurse training. Mental health nurses are in short supply and a bursary is given during training. Your experience in care will stand you in good stead and upon qualification you will be in a very good position to influence the standards of care for people with dementia and the training of future staff.

There are career prospects in care home management and as nurses working on wards and increasingly supporting older people with dementia and their carers in the community.

You owe it to yourself to consider it: talk to your nearest school of nursing.

Resources

Other resources

For activity and reminiscence material the following will be useful sources:

- *Libraries* – These are an obvious resource. Your local library will have books and other resources on themes which will be invaluable sources of quiz and reminiscence material. Most libraries also have a local history section which is a source of local reminiscence material, such as old newspapers and books showing how your local town has changed over the years. Libraries also have book sales on a regular basis as they upgrade their stock and this is a useful source of cheap material. Talk to the librarian about your needs.

- *Travel agents* – this is another excellent source of large colour photographs useful for reminiscence purposes. You should be raiding your local travel agents at least once or twice a year, but it is also worth while taking the time to explain what you want the pictures for. Tell them about reminiscence and see if they can help you out with large posters.

- *Contacts* – you should seek out the local branch of both the Alzheimer's Society and Age Concern.

Age Concern England
Astral House
1268 London Road
London SW16 4ER
Tel: 0208 765 7000
Ace@ace.org.uk
www.ageconcern.org.uk

Alzheimer's Society
Gordon Street
10 Greencoat Place
London SW1P 1PH
Tel: 0207 306 0606
Enquiries@alzheimers.org.uk
www.alzheimers.org.uk

Carers UK
20–25 Glasshouse Yard
London EC1A 4JT
Tel: 0207 490 8818
info@carersuk.org
www.carersuk.org

Centre for Policy on Ageing
25–31 Ironmonger Row
London EC1V 3QP
Tel: 0207 553 6500
cpa@cpa.org.uk
www.cpa.org.uk

Commission for Social Care Inspection
33 Greycoat Street
London SW1P 2QF
Tel: 0207 979 2000
enquiries@csci.gsi.gov.uk

Dementia Services Development Centre
University of Stirling
Stirling FK9 4LA
Scotland
Tel: 01786 467695
Dement1@stir.ac.uk
www.dsdc.stir.ac.uk

Department of Health
Richmond House
79 Whitehall
London SW1A 2NL
Tel: 0207 210 4850
dhmail@dh.gsi.gov.uk
www.dh.gov.uk

Help the Aged
207–221 Pentonville Road
London N1 9UZ
Tel: 0207 278 1114
info@helptheaged.org.uk
www.helptheaged.org.uk

Mind (National Association for Mental Health)
15–19 Broadway
London E15 4BQ
Tel: 0208 519 2122
contact@mind.org.uk
www.mind.org.uk

TOPSS (Training Organisation for the Personal Social Services)
26 Park Row
Leeds LS1 5QB
Tel: 0113 245 1716
info@topssengland.org.uk
www.topss.org.uk

Index

Lightning Source UK Ltd.
Milton Keynes UK
12 December 2010

164189UK00001B/22/P